Early years nutrition and healthy weight

EDITED BY

Dr Laura Stewart PhD, BSc, BA(HONS), RD

Joyce Thompson MPH, BSc, RD

WILEY Blackwell

This edition first published 2015 © 2015 by John Wiley & Sons, Ltd

Registered Office
John Wiley & Sons, Ltd, The Atrium, Southern Gate, Chichester, West Sussex, PO19 8SQ, UK

Editorial Offices
9600 Garsington Road, Oxford, OX4 2DQ, UK
The Atrium, Southern Gate, Chichester, West Sussex, PO19 8SQ, UK
350 Main Street, Malden, MA 02148-5020, USA

For details of our global editorial offices, for customer services and for information about how to apply for permission to reuse the copyright material in this book please see our website at www.wiley.com/wiley-blackwell

Library of Congress Cataloging-in-Publication Data

Early years nutrition and healthy weight / [edited by] Dr Laura Stewart, Joyce Thompson.
  p. ; cm.
 Includes bibliographical references and index.
 ISBN 978-1-118-79244-5 (pbk.)
I. Stewart, Laura, 1962– , editor.   II. Thompson, Joyce, 1959– , editor.
 [DNLM: 1. Child Nutritional Physiological Phenomena. 2. Pediatric Obesity. WS 130]
 RJ206
 613'.0432–dc23

                                2014035658

A catalogue record for this book is available from the British Library.

Wiley also publishes its books in a variety of electronic formats. Some content that appears in print may not be available in electronic books.

Cover image: iStockPhoto / © Patrick Heagney

Set in 9.5/12pt Meridien by SPi Publisher Services, Pondicherry, India

Printed in Singapore by C.O.S. Printers Pte Ltd

1   2015

Editors

Dr Laura Stewart PhD, BSc, BA(HONS), RD

Laura Stewart works for NHS Tayside in Scotland, UK. She is the Tayside Weight Management Pathway Manager, managing both adult and childhood obesity, while clinically specialising in childhood weight management. Laura graduated with a degree in Dietetics from Queen Margaret University, Edinburgh, in the early 1980s and has worked for the UK NHS since that time. She was a member of the Scottish Intercollegiate Guideline Network (SIGN) working groups on obesity for SIGN 69 (2003) and SIGN 115 (2010). She is a past chair of the British Dietetic Association's interest group Dietitians in Obesity Management UK (DOM UK). In 2014, Laura was a member of an Expert Group on childhood obesity which was set up to advise the Scottish Government.

Joyce Thompson MPH, BSc, RD

Joyce Thompson is a registered dietitian and works for NHS Tayside in Scotland. She was appointed as the Dietetic Consultant in Public Health Nutrition in 2004, Scotland's first Allied Health Profession consultant post. Joyce graduated with a degree in Dietetics from Queen Margaret University, Edinburgh, in 1982. She co-founded DOM UK and became its first chairperson. Joyce chaired the SIGN working group on obesity for SIGN 115 (2010).

Contents

Contributors

Louise A. Baur, AM, MBBS (Hons), BSc (Med), PhD, FRACP
Discipline of Paediatrics & Child Health, University of Sydney, Australia and
Weight Management Services, The Children's Hospital at Westmead, Westmead, Australia

Ethan A. Bergman, PhD, RDN, CD, FADA
Department of Nutrition, Exercise, and Health Sciences, College of Education and Professional
Studies, Academy of Nutrition and Dietetics, Central Washington University, Ellensburg, USA

Tracy Burrows, PhD, BHSc (N&D), AdvAPD
Priority Research Centre in Physical Activity and Nutrition, Faculty of Health and Medicine, The
University of Newcastle, Callaghan, Australia

Paul Chadwick, DClinPsy
Research Department of Clinical, Educational and Health Psychology, University College
London, London, UK

Clare Collins, PhD, BSc, Dip Nutr&Diet, Dip Clin Epi, FDAA
Priority Research Centre in Physical Activity and Nutrition, Faculty of Health and Medicine,
The University of Newcastle, Callaghan, Australia

Helen Croker, PhD, RD
Department of Epidemiology and Public Health, University College London, London, UK

Kerith Duncanson, BSc, Grad Dip (N&D), APD
Priority Research Centre in Physical Activity and Nutrition, Faculty of Health and Medicine,
The University of Newcastle, Callaghan, Australia

Catherine R. Hankey, PhD, SRD
Human Nutrition, University of Glasgow, Glasgow, UK

Adrienne R. Hughes, PhD
Physical Activity for Health Group, School of Psychological Sciences & Health, University of
Strathclyde, Glasgow, UK

Xanne Janssen, PhD
Physical Activity for Health Group, School of Psychological Sciences & Health, University of
Strathclyde, Glasgow, UK

Judy More, BSc, RD RNutr.
School of Health Professions, Plymouth University, Plymouth, UK and
Child-nutrition.co.uk Ltd, London, UK

Anthony D. Okely, EdD
Early Start Research Institute, University of Wollongong, Wollongong, Australia

John J. Reilly, PhD
Physical Activity for Health Group, School of Psychological Sciences & Health, University of Strathclyde, Glasgow, UK

Pinki Sahota, PhD
School of Health and Wellbeing, Leeds Beckett University, Leeds, UK

Charlotte M. Wright, B Med Sci, BMBCH, MSc, MD
Department of Child Health, School of Medicine, University of Glasgow, Glasgow, UK

Foreword

Childhood obesity is among the most common of chronic diseases and potentially one of the most preventable. Recent data from the USA suggests that although approximately 15% of pre-school children were overweight before they completed kindergarten, or when they were approximately 5.6 years of age, incidence of obesity in this group accounted for almost half of obesity present in 14-year-old adolescents [1]. In addition, although increased birth weight occurred in 12% of infants in this cohort, adolescents with increased birth weight accounted for over one-third of obesity present in 14-year-olds. These observations emphasize that successful, early efforts to prevent obesity in pre-school children or to successfully treat young children who are overweight or obese may be one of the most cost-effective strategies to reduce childhood obesity.

Two important repeated US cross-sectional studies suggest that increased awareness and changes in the consumption of high caloric density foods may already have begun to reduce the prevalence of obesity in pre-school-aged children. The Pediatric Nutrition Surveillance System (PedNSS) is an annual state-based survey of low-income children, most of whom are enrolled in the Women, Infants, and Children (WIC) food supplementation program. Between 2008 and 2011, the prevalence of obesity among several million 2–4-year-old children enrolled in PedNSS decreased in 18 states by approximately 5% (range 2–11%) [2]. Additional data from approximately 900 2–5-year-olds studied in the National Health and Nutrition Examination Survey (NHANES) reported a decrease of approximately 40% between 2004 and 2012 [3]. However, if that report had included earlier data from NHANES, the decrease would have been less dramatic.

The mechanism that can account for the decrease in prevalence in the USA can be understood in terms of the modest caloric deficits necessary to prevent obesity in young children. For example, the caloric deficits necessary to return the mean body mass index (BMI) to its 1970s level by the year 2020 is approximately 30 kcal/day for 2–5-year-olds, 150 kcal/day for 6–11-year-olds, and 180 kcal/day for 12–19-year-olds [4]. The decreases in early childhood obesity in the USA coincide with a number of shifts in the food supply and the consumption of high caloric density foods. The Healthy Weight Commitment Foundation is a group of food companies that supply approximately 25% of the calories in the USA. In 2010, these companies announced an effort to reduce the calories they provided by 1.5 trillion calories by 2015. Early in 2014, the companies announced that they had reduced the caloric content of their foods by 6.4 trillion calories, or approximately 78 kcal/person [5]. In addition, calories consumed from two of the leading sources of calories in the diets of children also declined. Energy from sugar drinks, which include colas and 10% juices, decreased by 37 kcal/day among 2–5-year-old US children [6], and fast food consumption decreased by 72 kcal/day among 2–11-year-old children [7].

These observations emphasize the importance and timeliness of a textbook devoted to the problem of obesity in young children. It is particularly appropriate to include the prenatal period, insofar as pre-pregnant weight, and excessive weight gain, tobacco use, and diabetes during pregnancy are all associated with early childhood obesity. A focus on risk factors in early childhood, such as the consumption of sugar drinks, fast food, and inactivity, is critical, in view of the growing appreciation of the effect of early onset of overweight on subsequent obesity. Although parenting is the final common pathway for these behaviors and their modification, only limited information exists regarding the parenting practices that predispose to childhood obesity and even less information on how to modify those behaviors. Finally, efforts to change the environment in places where children spend time, such as schools and child care centers, offer exceptionally promising loci for interventions, especially policy or regulatory strategies that increase the availability of low caloric density foods, reduce access to sugar drinks, mandate physical activity and limit screen time.

Although the caloric gap that can be achieved through policy changes in schools and child care will effectively prevent obesity, it will not likely be of sufficient magnitude to reduce body weight in those children who have already developed obesity. More rigorous clinical interventions will be required for this group. The development of effective clinical strategies for weight reduction will be even more challenging than the implementation of school and child care policies because physicians are poorly trained in how to begin a nonjudgmental conversation with families about their child's weight and in techniques to change behavior. In addition, a problem as prevalent as childhood obesity will require substantial changes in the care delivery system, with reliance on clinicians other than physicians. Changes in how care is delivered will also require additional adjustments on the part of physicians, who will need to learn how to work with other care providers. Finally, clinical interventions without changes in the environment will not likely sustain prevention or sustain weight loss after it occurs.

This text effectively addresses many of these areas and its authors are experts in the field. Our hope is that the lessons learned from its reading will inspire action and can be effectively implemented to reduce the prevalence and virulence of childhood obesity.

References

1 Cunningham SA, Kramer MR, Narayan KMV. Incidence of childhood obesity in the United States. *N Engl J Med* 2014; **370**(5): 403–11.
2 May AL, Pan L, Sherry B, Blanck HM, Galuska D, Dalenius K, Polhamus B, Kettel-Khan L, Grummer-Strawn LM. Vital signs: obesity among low-income, preschool-aged children – United States, 2008–2011. *Morbidity and Mortality Weekly Report* August 6, 2013; **62**: 1–6.
3 Ogden CL, Carroll MD, Kit BK, Flegal KM. Prevalence of childhood and adult obesity in the United States, 2011–2012. *JAMA* 2014; **311**(8): 806–14.
4 Wang YC, Orleans CT, Gortmaker SL. Reaching the healthy people goals for reducing childhood obesity: closing the energy gap. *Am J Prev Med* 2012; **42**(5): 437–44.
5 Robert Wood Johnson Foundation. *Major Food, Beverage Companies Remove 6.4 Trillion Calories from U.S. Marketplace*. January 9, 2014.
6 Kit BK, Fakhouri TH, Park S, Nielsen SJ, Ogden CL. Trends in sugar-sweetened beverage consumption among youth and adults in the United States: 1999–2010. *Am J Clin Nutr* 2013; **98**(1): 180–8.
7 Powell LM, Nguyen BT, Han E. Energy intake from restaurants: demographics and socioeconomics, 2003–2008. *Am J Prev Med* 2012; **43**(5): 498–504.

William H. Dietz MD, PhD
Director, Sumner M. Redstone Global Center on Prevention and Wellness,
Milken Institute School of Public Health
George Washington University,
Washington, DC

Acknowledgments

The editors, Laura Stewart and Joyce Thompson, would like to offer grateful appreciation and thanks to David Stewart, Kirsten Cumming and Sue Smart for their help with editing this book.

CHAPTER 1

Importance of good health and nutrition before and during pregnancy

Catherine R. Hankey

Human Nutrition, University of Glasgow, Glasgow, UK

Introduction

Pregnancy is a time of anticipation and excitement, especially for healthy mothers with no known health concerns for their foetus. It is increasingly evident that the lifestyle and health practices of mothers can impact markedly on their own health and that of their foetus.

Historically, pregnancy has been associated with 'blooming maternal health' and is probably the only period across the life course when positive encouragement for weight gain is given by many, at least in the developed world. Increasingly, given the world-wide epidemic of obesity, this positive response to sometimes excessive weight gain in pregnancy has been less widely accepted, but it does still have cross-cultural impact. Pregnancy can also offer a positive setting which may increase the willingness of the individual to consider improving their health. It has been envisaged as a 'new start', which has been associated with positive improvements in lifestyle. Research has examined whether pregnant women can be encouraged to become more physically active, to attempt smoking cessation and to minimise or avoid alcohol intake. Attempts have been made to alter women's food choice during pregnancy towards eating more healthy foods such as fruit and vegetables, and away from foods rich in fat and sugar which have often been associated with negative health consequences including the development of gestational diabetes (GDM). Good maternal health both pre-conceptually and during pregnancy has long been recognised as valuable. Evidence is accruing that preparing for pregnancy could offer real health benefits to both maternal and infant health, particularly in the context of the current obesity epidemic. However, this opportunity appears only available to few; for example in the UK, only around 50% of all pregnancies are reported as planned and there were close to 800 000 live births in 2012 [1].

Importance of good maternal health before and during pregnancy

Good maternal health is crucial to reduce the chances of adverse outcomes such as GDM, miscarriage, pre-eclampisa, still birth, macrosomia and caesarean section for the mother, and abnormal birth weight and increased risk of obesity in infancy for the unborn child.

Early Years Nutrition and Healthy Weight, First Edition. Edited by Laura Stewart and Joyce Thompson.
© 2015 John Wiley & Sons, Ltd. Published 2015 by John Wiley & Sons, Ltd.

Abstinence from smoking and alcohol consumption together with regular physical activity has long been advocated to pregnant women, given the benefits this can bring for maternal and foetal health. Maternal nutritional status has been recognised as important before and during pregnancy, to maximise the chances of a healthy pregnancy and an optimal outcome for both mother and infant. Historically, dietary advice for optimal health in pregnancy has focussed on healthy eating with an emphasis on the maintenance of good health in terms of dietary intakes, and a sufficient intake of macro- and micro-nutrients [2]. Dietary advice advocated for all adults and appropriate to pregnant women to increase awareness and encourage them to eat well is illustrated in the UK's visual representation 'The Eatwell Plate' [3] (see Chapter 8). This graphic representation, designed for use by all adults, appears to have achieved consensus as a valuable tool, and as well as due to its widespread use in UK National Health Service (NHS), it is advocated by various health charities. However, uncertainties remain as to the scientific evidence on which the tool's graphic representation is based.

It has recently been highlighted that most pregnant women want to know the best foods to eat and what they should avoid. Current issues of concern include the possible dangers of eating liver, the need to avoid unprocessed cheese and too much tuna and oil-rich fish beyond two portions per week [4, 5].

According to National Institute of Health and Care Excellence (NICE), alcohol, for those in the first 12 weeks of pregnancy, should be avoided completely, and intakes throughout the remainder of pregnancy ought to be very limited, due to potential negative effects on foetal health [6]. Furthermore, as alcohol supplies energy of 7 kcal/g, it is considered as a concentrated source of energy, and hence even moderate consumption may increase energy intakes and encourage excessive prenatal weight gain.

Maternal caffeine intake has received considerable interest, given suggestions that raised intakes increase the likelihood of foetal growth restriction. In a large prospective observational study in two UK maternity units [7], retrospective caffeine intakes were determined and findings indicated that low caffeine intakes (up to 100 mg/day) are safe, but higher levels, in excess of 200 mg/day, increased the risk of miscarriage, premature birth and low birth–weight babies. Two hundred milligram of caffeine equates to around two cups daily of tea and/or coffee, though other rich sources such as caffeinated drinks should also be considered. Decaffeinated versions of these drinks may be of value.

Link between maternal diet and foetal growth

Dietary patterns in pregnancy have been studied using factor analyses or similar component analyses to investigate links between maternal diet and foetal growth, and dietary patterns in pregnancy and their associations with socioeconomic status (SES) and lifestyle. This is arguably a clear way to examine diet and health relationships, as the human diet contains a wide variety of nutrients and many may correlate with health outcomes. Danish researchers looked at associations between dietary patterns and foetal growth in over 40 000 pregnant women. Three major dietary patterns were observed: (1) a western diet rich in dairy fat and red and processed meats, (2) a healthy diet rich in fruit, vegetables, poultry and fish and (3) a mixture of both. The health conscious pattern was associated with a 24% lower occurrence of a small for gestational age (SGA) babies [8]. This pattern was evident when parity, maternal smoking, age, height, pre-pregnancy weight and fathers' height were included as confounding factors.

Using the Avon Longitudinal Study of Parents and Children (ALSPAC) data [9], Northstone *et al.* examined dietary patterns in the third trimester of pregnancy. Associations were determined between social and demographic characteristics and habitual dietary intake when estimated using a food frequency questionnaire. Dietary patterns were categorised into four broad groups: (1) 'processed diet', full of high fat foods, (2) the 'confectionary diet', (3) the 'vegetarian diet' and (4) the 'health conscious diet' where the latter dietary pattern fulfilled the majority of dietary targets and was favoured by educated, older and non-white pregnant mothers.

In contrast, poorer diets were favoured by pregnant woman who smoked and were white, young and overweight.

Whilst ALSPAC data indicated the associations between dietary patterns and characteristics of the pregnant women, the Danish study illustrated a positive link between poorer dietary patterns and SGA babies, when the socio-economic and other factors were controlled. This epidemiological evidence favours specific macronutrients or micronutrients that may be underlying the association with SGA.

Micronutrients most likely to be at risk in pregnancy

The micronutrients most commonly at risk of shortfalls are iron, vitamin D and folic acid. A recent systematic review confirmed that in the UK and other developed countries, intakes of all these micronutrients are consistently reported to be below national recommendations [10]. The accuracy of these findings has been compromised by the limitations of dietary intake measurements, but a clear trend towards suboptimal intakes is evident. For these reasons, this chapter will deliberately focus on these key micronutrients.

Iron

Recent estimates, according to the Nutrition Impact Model Study, of the worldwide prevalence of anaemia in pregnant women is 38% (95% CI 33–43), that is 32 (28–36) million pregnant women globally [11]. Anaemia in pregnancy, diagnosed using World Health Organization (WHO) guidance [12], is defined as a haemoglobin concentration less than 11.0 g/l. Around 50% of anaemia is estimated to be as a result of iron deficiency, the world's most commonly occurring nutritional disorder. Inadequate iron intakes are known to compromise maternal and foetal well-being, and intervention strategies to manage the situation should be implemented. This usually comes in the form of dietary advice, but more common is iron supplementation.

Dietary approaches to managing iron status

Advice given in antenatal clinics should be appropriate with respect to iron status. The UK Scientific Advisory Committee on Nutrition (SACN) has recently summarised its guidance on how to challenge a shortfall in iron status: 'a healthy balanced diet', which includes a variety of foods containing iron, will help people achieve adequate iron status [13]. Such an approach is more effective than consuming iron-rich foods at the same time as foods/drinks that enhance iron absorption (e.g. citrus fruit juice, red meat) whilst avoiding foods containing components that inhibit iron absorption (e.g. tea, coffee, milk).

Given the increasing concern that one of the major sources of dietary iron – red and processed meat products – has been linked to the development of colon cancer, the SACN report indicated that intakes of red and processed meat, which they considered high, ≥90 g/day should be reduced by at least 20% to a total intake of 70 g/day cooked weight. The committee considered that reducing red meat intakes by this magnitude would not compromise iron status in those of the adult population with low intakes but could beneficially affect colon cancer risk.

The risk of compromised iron status is increased in pregnancy, given its additional iron requirements. Iron requirements increase across pregnancy, reaching 30 mg/day during the final trimester. In order to help satisfy these increased needs, the proportion of iron which is absorbed in pregnant woman is increased from around 15% of all consumed to up to 45%. Education and counselling regarding diet may improve iron intake and enhance absorption but the degree of change achievable, especially in 'hard to reach' individuals, such as those living in deprivation, ethnic minorities, etc. remains in doubt.

How effective are iron supplements in pregnancy?

The effectiveness of iron supplements in pregnancy for those with anaemia has recently been evaluated in a systematic review and meta-analysis [14]. This review used international data to summarise the available evidence on the associations of maternal anaemia and prenatal iron use with maternal haematology and adverse pregnancy outcomes. Any relationships between exposure and response were examined such as between dose of iron, duration of use and haemoglobin concentration in the prenatal period, with pregnancy outcomes. Daily prenatal use of iron substantially improved prenatal mean haemoglobin concentrations. The authors concluded that given the worldwide prevalence of anaemia and iron deficiency, they considered it justified to expose an entire population (i.e. all pregnant women) to iron supplementation. As iron deficiency is a preventable disease for which cost-effective treatment is easy to administer, they felt justified in their conclusions. A Cochrane review [15] also concluded that prenatal daily or weekly iron supplementation was effective in reducing the risk of low birth–weight babies and in preventing maternal anaemia and iron deficiency. Iron absorption is physiologically regulated and relies on the natural mechanism regulating total body iron; therefore, it should protect against iron overload. Side effects, and hence poor compliance, can be relieved by administration of the iron supplements with food, although this may decrease absorption, particularly of ferrous preparations.

Iron supplementation to all 'healthy' pregnant women

In contrast to the views detailed earlier, it has been recommended that routine iron supplementation is unjustified in 'healthy' pregnant women [16]. Their argument is twofold. Firstly, the number of hazards associated with iron supplementation, not least that the preparation can be toxic, and oral iron supplements often have gastrointestinal side effects, which are unpleasant. Therefore exposing an entire population to excess iron is unjustified and should not take place without good reason. Secondly, the case for oral iron supplementation should ideally be guided by early or pre-pregnancy ferritin measurements. The view taken by NICE [6] and the British Committee for Standards in Haematology [17] is that iron status in pregnancy ought to be reviewed routinely, and all women should have a full blood count taken at the booking appointment (week 12 of pregnancy) and at 28 weeks [6]. This should facilitate selective iron supplementation early in pregnancy, although effective systems must be in place for rapid review of blood results and appropriate follow-up.

In the UK, pregnant women with a haemoglobin level less than 11 g/l up until 12 weeks or less than 10.5 g/l beyond 12 weeks should be offered a trial of therapeutic iron replacement. In non-anaemic women at increased risk of iron depletion, including those with previous anaemia, multiple pregnancy or consecutive pregnancies with less than a year's interval between and vegetarians, a serum ferritin measurement (the best indicator of maternal iron stores) should be considered. If the ferritin level is less than 30 µg/l, then 65 mg elemental iron once a day should be offered [17].

Vitamin D

Inadequate vitamin D status is becoming increasingly common in pregnant women. Those with coloured skin, who live in cool climates where sunlight levels are limited and insufficient to allow vitamin D to be synthesised in the skin, are especially vulnerable. Covering of almost all skin, sometimes leaving only the eyes visible as evident in devout religious women leads to poor vitamin D status, especially in a temperate climate such as the UK. The occurrence of infantile rickets is increasing and highlights the need for provision of vitamin D supplements to all those at risk of poor vitamin D status in pregnancy. To meet this goal, 10 µg daily supplementation of vitamin D is advocated throughout pregnancy [6, 18] with a need for clinicians to be especially vigilant towards the vitamin D status of women from black and ethnic minorities, the socially excluded, those with limited exposure to sunlight and the obese (pre-pregnancy body mass index (BMI) >30 kg/m^2). The latter group is considered to be susceptible to vitamin D deficiency due to the sequestration of vitamin D into adipose tissue, rather than liver sites, where it then becomes unavailable [19]. Despite the additional requirements of pregnancy, there is insufficient evidence to advocate increasing the daily 10 µg vitamin D supplement level [18].

Folic acid supplementation to prevent neural tube defects

In 1991, folic acid supplementation among women planning a pregnancy was shown to prevent a proportion of neural tube defects (NTD) [20] and the evidence was overwhelming; national authorities such as the health departments for England, Wales and Scotland each have a consensus recommendation that all women planning a pregnancy should increase their intake of folic acid. The recommended folic acid intake is about double the current estimated dietary intake of 0.2 mg/day [21], though the mechanism of action is unclear.

As with vitamin D, there have been suggestions that higher levels of folate supplements are required for obese pregnant mother. These larger supplemental doses are required for a number of reasons, for example a higher risk of NTD in the obese; odds ratios for an NTD-affected pregnancy are 1.22 (95% CI 0.99–1.49), 1.70 (95% CI 1.34–2.15) and 3.11 (95% CI 1.75–5.46) for women defined as overweight, obese and severely obese respectively [22]. Folate status is shown to be lower in obese adults than in healthy normal weight adults probably due to a poor quality of diet , and it has been shown that a 0.2 µg dosage of folic acid has a lower impact reflected in lower plasma concentrations in obese adults than in healthy normal weight adult. However, a rate of supplementation guided by BMI may be justified by cogent research findings.

Nevertheless, despite guidance by leading expert committees in the fields of obstetrics and gynaecology [23], the folic acid dosage for the obese remains at 0.2 μg/day rather than at 5 μg/day, as advocated by this guideline.

From a public health perspective, NTD affects only a minority of people at risk, hence, there is a dilemma over the widespread use of folic acid supplementation in flour and other food stuff. USA data report NTD incidence at about 3.5 cases per 10 000 births, a fall from 5 cases prior to the widespread use of prenatal folic acid supplementation. However, given the need for folic acid to be ideally consumed pre-conceptually, and at least up until the first 12 weeks of pregnancy, potentially many women do not comply with supplements. One approach to resolve this issue would be mandatory fortification of flour with folic acid, which currently occurs in over 70 countries worldwide but not in the UK.

Factors associated with poor uptake of folic acid supplements are perhaps predictable and include educating those individuals. An initiative in the north of the Netherlands resulted in 51% women using folic acid supplements appropriately [24]. The socio-demographic and lifestyle factors associated with non-compliance with pre-conceptual use of folic acid included non-western ethnicity, and not having a partner. Fortification of staple foods with folic acid would provide a more effective means of ensuring an adequate intake, especially for those groups of women who are unlikely to plan their pregnancies or to receive and respond to health promotion messages.

The SACN committee [25] believes that sufficient evidence exists to proceed with fortification of flour with folic acid, though the issue still remains under consideration. This is despite some apparent associations between excess folic acid intake and the incidence of colon cancer, although the epidemiological data to date remain inconclusive. However, as with any large public health initiative, consideration of other population groups is required, before implementation. In this case, in order to avoid exposing groups of the population to higher than recommended doses of folic acid, voluntary supplementation of foods with folic acid should be prevented, prior to any country wide fortification.

Weight gain in pregnancy: what is optimal and how can this weight change be judged?

Given the widespread increase in the prevalence of overweight and obesity, with greater numbers of women affected than men, specific guidelines for optimal weight gain throughout pregnancy are justified. UK data report a doubling of maternal obesity from 7.6 to 15.6% between 1989 and 2007 [26], an observation which has now been replicated across the developed world. The United States (US) Institute of Medicine

Table 1.1 United States Institute of Medicine guideline weights for maternal weight gain according to BMI*.

Pre-pregnancy BMI	BMI (kg/m²) (WHO)	Total weight gain range (lbs)	Rates of weight gain second and third trimester (mean range in lbs/week)
Underweight	<18.5	28–40	1 (1–1.3)
Normal weight	18.5–24.9	25–35	1 (0.8–1)
Overweight	25.0–29.9	15–25	0.6 (0.5–0.7)
Obese (includes all classes)	≥30.0	11–20	0.5 (0.4–0.6)

* Reproduced with permission from Ref. 27. © Nature Publishing Group.

(IOM) launched revised guidelines [27], and given a dearth of others, these guidelines appear the most widely recognised and used internationally. The guidelines are based on observational studies, but importantly the weight gain referred to is not just due to increased adipose tissue but also the placenta, foetus and associated tissues. The IOM clearly recognised the need for BMI specific weight gain guidance, and these are increasingly used in clinical practice internationally (Table 1.1).

Why is excessive gestational weight gain a concern in pregnancy?

The presence of obesity and to a lesser extent overweight is the most common obstetric issue in the developed world. There are numerous negative health consequences, more evident in the case of obesity that can affect the health of both mother and foetus. These include GDM and pre-eclampsia in the mother and the risks of babies born large or those SGA. The implications of excessive weight gain are considerable, and in the case of GDM may persist into future generations. Fertility is compromised by raised BMI, and this may reduce the likelihood of future pregnancies in the obese mother [28]. The birthing process itself is also often compromised in the obese, with induction of labour, and high levels of intervention required more frequently than in non-obese women. Recent analyses have indicated that even moderate elevations in maternal BMI were associated with a 20% increased risk of foetal death. It should be noted, however, that this study may indicate a worse-case scenario as the comparator to estimate risk was a BMI of 20kg/m^2 [2, 29].

Many consider pregnancy as a period in the life course which favours weight retention post-natally leading to both overweight and obesity. In response, research interest has focused on the development of interventions to challenge this persistent problem, and ideally such interventions should be implemented pre-conceptually.

Pre-conception interventions

Given the fact that pregnancy imposes physiological stress which is often elevated in proportion to BMI, one solution could be a pre-pregnancy intervention to improve the health and fertility of women pre-conceptually. Whilst a prenatally delivered intervention may offer significant benefits, this is an area which is challenging to address. The lack of evidence in this area reflects these difficulties with the feasibility of any prenatal intervention. Challenges are likely to include identifying women who are planning a pregnancy, and willing to postpone their attempts at conception, until their weight has been reduced. A recent study [30] delivered using the internet was moderately successful in women who were preparing for pregnancy. Despite an attrition rate of close to 55% after the 6 month intervention, an improvement in favourable behaviours was reported. A decrease in alcohol intakes and an increase in compliance with folic acid supplementation was reported, although interestingly no impact on BMI or smoking habits was evident. In general, there was an improvement in the knowledge of participants concerning pre-conceptual health to avoid adverse pregnancy outcomes was shown but this was not universal. The women who completed the programme were more likely to be graduates who were in employment, perhaps suggesting a suitability of these sectors of society to this style of intervention. This framework is attractive and offers promise to identify those considering pregnancy and improve their preparation for this. As such this area deserves further evaluation.

Current practice

According to IOM guidelines, the aim for a pregnant woman who is obese is to minimise their gestational weight gain. However, counter intuitively, current UK practice is not to weigh pregnant women beyond their week 12 booking appointment. The pros and cons of regular weighing throughout pregnancy have been considered but at present regular weighing is only advocated for those at risk of insufficient weight gain, which may compromise a pregnancy and baby weight. NICE do not advocate regular weighing, and at present, there is no evidence from randomised controlled trials to support its use.

Health professionals who deliver antenatal care appear the obvious candidates to expand their routine contacts to address issues associated with weight issues. This is particularly true given the mounting evidence to link high weight gains with development of GDM among other negative maternal and foetal health consequences [31]. Midwives have reported unease about raising the issue of a women's weight during their consultations. The reasons commonly reported in UK and Australian studies relate to compromising their clinical relationship with their patient and feeling insufficiently trained to manage any weight-related issues [32, 33].

Furthermore, many pregnant women report being unconcerned about their weight gain in pregnancy, despite many having already gained weight in previous pregnancies and failed to return to their pre-pregnancy weight [34]. This study found over 80% of participants expressed dissatisfaction with their current weight but were still resistant to dietary strategies to avoid excessive weight gain. They reported a preference for increasing their physical activity which they recognised as being valuable in pregnancy [35]. However, it is likely that self-assessment of fitness levels is unrealistic and the feasibility of undertaking through increased activity is unrealistic, especially as their pregnancy progressed. It may indirectly suggest that overweight pregnant woman either felt they had sufficient knowledge of 'healthy eating' or considered pregnancy a time when self imposed restrained eating to limit weight may be not required.

Impact of pregnancy and breast feeding on energy requirements

The myth that a pregnant woman is actually eating for two is an old one, probably first becoming popular in times of food scarcity. In actual fact, there is only a small increase in energy requirements in pregnancy, largely in the third trimester. This is estimated at around 191 kcal/day, when weight gain is most rapid. For those who choose to breastfeed and are able to do so, the additional energy needs for lactation are close to 502 kcal/day. These estimates are based on requirements for those whose BMI is in excess or below the midpoint BMI of 22.5 kg/m^2 [2, 36]. Whilst it is recognised that breastfeeding has great benefits for maternal and infant health, and should be advocated in all cases, its role in offering benefits in weight control is unclear. It is difficult to distinguish from other factors predicting maternal weight loss post-natally such as low junk food intake, regular physical activity, healthy food choices and hormonal contraception [37].

Underweight and pregnancy outcome

Being of a low BMI (<18.5 kg/m²) has been shown to be a risk factor for poor pregnancy outcome. It is strongly associated with poor or suboptimal fertility and impacts on neonatal health, particularly increased morbidity and mortality risks associated with preterm birth. A low BMI is one of the few modifiable risk factors. However, a cohort study indicated that to undergo large fluctuations in BMI prior to pregnancy has an increased risk of premature birth, a risk higher in someone who had already experienced a pre-term birth [38]. The potential value of pre-conceptual care may be evident in the setting of undernutrition.

Gestational weight gain (GWG) is known to have mixed effects on post-natal health. ALSPAC data have shown that those with low GWG during pregnancy also had a lower initial BMI than those who gained weight as recommended or who exceeded weight gain guidelines. These findings indicate that managing and optimising pre-pregnancy weight may offer health benefits. GWG impacts differently on both mothers and babies and often shows contrasting associations [39].

How can the excessive GWG be challenged?

Given the recognised risks associated with being overweight or obese in pregnancy, there have been a number of studies which have looked at formal approaches to weight management. Weight management in pregnancy is different, and weight loss is not advocated [6]. A stalling of weight gain in the overweight and an increase in appropriate physical activity, such as walking etc., are the only tools that are available and safe to utilise.

Such an intervention was reported in a randomised controlled study in which women with a BMI of close to 35 kg/m² were recruited at 15 weeks gestation [40]. Treatment allocation was either to usual care or to a 10-hour one-to-one intervention delivered by a dietitian. Dietary advice focussed on, low fat food intakes which were eucaloric with the individuals estimated energy requirements. The intervention group minimised their GWG to approximately 7 kg, while the control group gained approximately 13 kg. Glucose metabolism was also superior to the control subjects and this was reflected in a lower glycated haemoglobin (HbA1c). Similar positive findings were seen in other small studies, including one which showed no negative effects from weight management which imposed a moderate energy deficit along with advice to take regular physical activity. Importantly, negative effects on breastfeeding and infant weight were observed, as this is something that practitioner's report as a potential disadvantage of weight management post-natally [41].

The recently completed randomised controlled LIMIT study appeared an idealised approach to challenge excessive maternal weight gain in obese or overweight pregnant women [42]. Comprehensive dietary advice and plans for appropriate physical activity were delivered using current guidelines and by experts to deliver and reinforce the advice. It was a light touch intervention which offered women with a singleton pregnancy whose BMI was $\geq 25\,kg/m^2$, guidance and support to minimise excessive weight gain. Primary outcome was the delivery of a baby over the 90th centile weight, with a number of relevant secondary outcomes covering maternal weight and co-morbidities, including delivery methods. Despite this comprehensive intervention, there were no reported differences in either group at birth. Upon reflection, the authors suggested that perhaps the intervention as delivered was insufficiently intensive or too 'light touch' and/or that alterations in lifestyle implemented by women were insufficient to impact on outcomes. It is hoped that the ongoing complex lifestyle intervention to challenge excessive GWG, the 'upbeat study' [43] will reduce occurrence of GDM and the birth of large for gestational age babies. It is clear that the roadmap to managing GWG, particularly in the obese and overweight, is challenging. The majority of interventions have failed to show clinically important benefits on maternal or infant outcomes resulting from lifestyle interventions. Also of concern is the pilot work that has shown that accessing those pregnant women who are at high risk of negative excess weight–related pregnancies who live in relative poverty can be even more difficult to achieve [44].

Conclusions

Nutritional advice is most often aimed at the pregnant women's dietary intake, with the aim of ensuring that she is consuming 'sufficient foods' from all of the different food groups to achieve the appropriate dietary references values [45] or SACN target [35]. There are opportunities to minimise energy intake, but within current clinical practice in the UK, there are no particular approaches that are regularly in use. Supplementation with folic acid and in many cases vitamin D is now securely supported by evidence; however, compliance with these supplements remains an issue for the more vulnerable in our society.

Prenatal care, such as initiating supplemental folic acid consumption and improving diet composition and reducing body weight where required, is an attractive option to maximise maternal and foetal health. However, the role of fortification of flour with folic acid appears a solution to accessing those in society who are reluctant to comply with supplementation.

All women with a $\geq$ BMI $30\,kg/m^2$ should be advised by a trained health professional of the benefits of healthy food habit and how this can best be put into practice. However, the impact of such advice is unclear, and given the increasing occurrence of obese and overweight pregnancy, it is probably fair to conclude that effects have been very limited. Robust evidence confirms the negative effects of obesity and overweight on maternal and foetal health. Management approaches pre-conceptually and post-natally following current guidelines are valuable; however, the major studies which have used robust study designs and comprehensive interventions to challenge excessive GWG have found only weak effects of the interventions at best. At present, there is insufficient evidence to incorporate these approaches in routine clinical practice.

Perhaps the period of pregnancy is too short to accommodate lifestyle change, given it is 12 weeks of pregnancy before pregnant women enter the care of the midwife and other professionals. It may be that the period between pregnancies is an avenue that can be pursued with new mothers being recruited when attending their post-natal baby checks.

CASE STUDY: AWARENESS OF OBESITY AND RISK TO HEALTH OF WOMEN AND UNBORN CHILD

Question: Current practice in antenatal care in the UK does not recommend regular weighing of women after a booking clinic weight is taken at week 12 or thereabout [6]. Many pregnant women are overweight, or even obese before conception, and often deny that there are any problems which may negatively affect their own and their baby's health.

You are a midwife faced with a very overweight pregnant lady. Her BMI at her 12 week booking clinic was greater than $35\,kg/m^2$, she is hypertensive without family history of pre-eclampsia and this is her first pregnancy. How should you best manage this patient to maximise the chances of a healthy pregnancy and live birth?

Answer:
1 Assess and monitor weight.
2 Aim to prevent excessive weight gain.
3 Support the woman to achieve and maintain an appropriate weight by eating healthily and regularly undertaking physical activity amenable to pregnancy.
- Advise that eating a balanced and healthy diet and being physically active during pregnancy will offer health benefits to both herself and her unborn child.
- Dispel any myths about what and how much to eat during pregnancy, explain that energy needs do not change in the first 6 months of pregnancy and increase little in the last 3 months (by around 200 kcal/day).
- Reputable advice and advice on diet is available to health professionals from NHS choices website, local public health and dietetic departments. NICE [6] indicates that practical and tailored information is considered most effective. This could be dietary advice concentrating on minimising high-calorie snacking and generally reducing overeating.
- Recommend increasing physical activity. Regular and moderate intensity exercise has been shown to be difficult for pregnant women to implement. The woman should be reassured that this activity will not harm her or her unborn child.
- At least 30 minutes/day of moderate intensity activity is recommended. Information should be as specific and tailored as possible to the individual. Recreational exercise such as swimming or brisk walking and strength conditioning exercise is safe and beneficial and most likely to be adhered to. Emphasise the aim is to stay fit, rather than to reach peak fitness. For those women who have not exercised routinely they should begin with not more than 15 minutes/day.
- Offer regular monitoring of weight changes and lifestyle management. This would ideally support any lifestyle changes and provide additional support. This could be the midwife herself or another professional who could support this.

References

1 Tommy's. *Pregnancy Research.* http://www.tommys.org/ (accessed 21 April 2014).
2 Anderson AS. Nutrition and pregnancy – motivations and interests. *J Hum Nutr Diet* 2003; **16**: 65–66.
3 Department of Health (2010). *Your Guide to the Eatwell Plate.* https://www.gov.uk/government/uploads/system/uploads/attachment_data/file/237282/Eatwell_plate_booklet.pdf (accessed 8 May 2014).
4 NHS Choices (2014). *Foods to Avoid in Pregnancy.* http://www.nhs.uk/conditions/pregnancy-and-baby/pages/foods-to-avoid-pregnant.aspx#close (accessed 8 May 2014).
5 Poston L. Healthy eating in pregnancy. Always a good idea, now with more supporting evidence. *BMJ* 2014; **348**: 1–2.
6 NICE (2008). *Antenatal Care NICE Clinical Guideline 62.* http://www.nice.org.uk/nicemedia/live/11947/40115/40115.pdf (accessed 12 May 2014).
7 CARE Study Group. Maternal caffeine intake during pregnancy and risk of fetal growth restriction: a large prospective observational study. *BMJ* 2008; **337**: 1–8.
8 Knudsen VK, Orozova-Bekkevold IM, Mikkelsen TB, Wolff S, Olsen SF. Major dietary patterns in pregnancy and foetal growth. *Eur J Clin Nutr* 2008; **62**: 463–470.
9 Northstone K, Emmett P, Roger I. Dietary patterns in pregnancy and associations with socio-demographic and lifestyle factors. *Eur J Clin Nutr* 2008; **62**: 471–479.

10 Blumfield ML, Collins C, MacDonald-Wicks L, Hure AJ, Smith R. A systematic reviews and meta-analysis of micronutrient intakes during pregnancy in developed countries. *Nutr Rev* 2013; **71**: 118–132.

11 Stevens G, Finucane M, De-Regil L, Paciorek C, Flaxman S, Branca F. Global, regional, and national trends in total and severe anaemia prevalence in children and pregnant and non-pregnant women. *Lancet Glob Health* 2013; **1**: 16–25.

12 World Health Organisation Reproductive Health Library (2007). *Treatments for Iron-Deficiency Anaemia in Pregnancy*. http://apps.who.int/rhl/pregnancy_childbirth/medical/anaemia/cfcom/en/ (accessed 12 May 2014).

13 Scientific Advisory Committee on Nutrition (2011). *SCAN Iron and Health Report*. http://www.sacn.gov.uk/reports_position_statements/reports/sacn_iron_and_health_report.html (accessed 21 April 2014).

14 Haider BA, Olofin I, Wang M, Spiegelman D, Ezzati M, Fawzi WW, on behalf of Nutrition Impact Model Study Group (anaemia). Anaemia, prenatal iron use, and risk of adverse pregnancy outcomes: systematic review and meta-analysis. *BMJ* 2013; **346**: 1–19.

15 Pena-Rosas JP, Viteri FE. Effects and safety of preventive oral iron or iron + folic acid supplementation for women during pregnancy. *Cochrane Database Syst Rev* 2009; **4**: CD004736.

16 Steer P. Healthy pregnant women still don't need routine iron supplementation. *BMJ* 2013; **347**: 1.

17 British Committee for Standards in Haematology (2012). *UK Guidelines on the Management of Iron Deficiency in Pregnancy*. http://www.bcshguidelines.com/documents/UK_Guidelines_iron_deficiency_in_pregnancy.pdf (accessed 13 May 2014).

18 Royal College of Obstetrician and Gynaecologists (2012). *RCOG Statement on Vitamin D Supplementation for Pregnant Women*. http://www.rcog.org.uk/what-we-do/campaigning-and-opinions/statement/rcog-statement-vitamin-d-supplementation-pregnant-wome (accessed 8 May 2014).

19 Wortsman J, Matsuoka LY, Chen TC, Lu Z, Holick MF. Decreased bioavailability of vitamin D in obesity. *Am J Clin Nutr* 2000; **72** (3): 690–693.

20 Medical Research Council Vitamin Study Research Group. Prevention of neural tube defects: results of the Medical Research Council vitamin study. *Lancet* 1991; **338**: 131–137.

21 Scientific Advisory Committee on Nutrition (2006). *Folate and Disease Prevention*. http://www.sacn.gov.uk/pdfs/folate_and_disease_prevention_report.pdf (accessed 8 May 2014).

22 Rasmussen SA, Chu SY, Kim SY, Schmid CH, Lau J. Maternal obesity and risk of neural tube defects. *Am J Obstet Gynecol* 2008; **198** (6): 611–619.

23 Royal College of Obstetrician and Gynaecologists (2010). *CMACE/ RCOG Joint Guideline: Management of Women with Obesity in Pregnancy*. http://www.hqip.org.uk/assets/NCAPOP-Library/CMACE-Reports/15.-March-2010-Management-of-Women-with-Obesity-in-Pregnancy-Guidance.pdf (accessed 21 April 2014).

24 Mannien J, de Jonge A, Cornel MC, Spelten E, Hutton EK. Factors associated with not using folic acid supplements pre-conceptionally. *Public Health Nutr* 2013; **10**: 1–7.

25 Scientific Advisory Committee on Nutrition (2009). *Folic Acid and Colorectal Cancer Risk: Review of Recommendation for Mandatory Folic Acid Fortification*. http://www.sacn.gov.uk/pdfs/summary_of_sacn_report_to_cmo_ 19_october_2009.pdf (accessed 8 May 2014).

26 Heslehurst N, Rankin J, Wilkinson JR, Summerbell CD. A nationally representative study of maternal obesity in England UK: trends in incidence and demographic inequalities in 619 323 births 1989–2007. *Int J Obes (Lond)* 2010; **34** (3): 420–428.

27 Institute of Medicine. *Weight Gain during Pregnancy: Re-examining the Guidelines*. http://iom.edu/~/media/Files/Report%20Files/2009/Weight-Gain-During-Pregnancy-Reexamining-the-Guidelines/Report%20Brief%20-%20Weight%20Gain%20During%20Pregnancy.pdf (accessed 13 May 2014).

28 Yazdani S, Yosofniyapasha Y, Nasab BH, Mojaveri MH, Bouzari Z (2009). Effect of maternal body mass index on pregnancy outcome and newborn weight. *BMC Res Notes* 2012; **5**: 34–38.

29 Dagfinn A, Saugstad O, Henriksen T, Tonstad S. Maternal body mass index and the risk of fetal death, stillbirth, and infant death: a systematic review and meta-analysis. *JAMA* 2014; **311** (15): 1536–1546.

30 Agricola E, Pandolfi E, Gonfiantini M, Gesualdo F, Romano M, Carloni E, *et al*. A cohort study of a tailored web intervention for preconception care. *BMC Med Inform Decis Mak* 2014; **14**: 1–10.

31 Sommer C, Morkrid K, Jenum AK, Sletner L, Mosdol A, Birkeland KI. Weight gain, total fat gain and regional fat gain during pregnancy and the association with gestational diabetes: a population based cohort study. *Int J Obes (Lond)* 2014; **38**: 76–81.

32 Heslehurst N, Russell S, McCormack S, Sedgewick G, Bell R, Rankin J. Midwives perspectives of their training and education requirements in maternal obesity: a qualitative study. *Midwifery* 2013; **29** (7): 736–744.

33 Knight-Agarwal CR, Kaur M, Williams LT, Davey R, Davis D. The views and attitudes of health professionals providing antenatal care to women with a high BMI: a qualitative research study. *Women Birth* 2014; **27** (2): 138–144.

34 Leslie WS, Gibson A, Hankey CR. Prevention and management of excessive gestational weight gain: a survey of overweight and obese pregnant women. *BMC Pregnancy Childbirth* 2013; **13** (10): 1–7.

35 Duckitt KL. Exercise during pregnancy, eat for one, exercise for two. *BMJ* 2011; **343**: 1–2.

36 Scientific Advisory Committee on Nutrition (2011). *Dietary Reference Values for Energy*. http://www.sacn.gov.uk/pdfs/sacn_dietary_reference_values_for_energy.pdf (accessed 12 May 2014).

37 Østbye T, Peterson BL, Krause KM, Swamy GK, Lovelady CA. Predictors of postpartum weight change among overweight and obese women: results from the Active Mothers Postpartum study. *J Womens Health* 2012; **21** (2): 215–222.

38 Merlino A, Laffineuse L, Collin M, Mercer B. Impact of weight loss between pregnancies on recurrent preterm birth. *Am J Obstet Gynecol* 2006; **195** (3): 818–821.

39 Fraser A, Tilling K, MacDonald-Wallis C, Sattar N, Brion MJ, Benfield L, *et al.* Association of maternal weight gain in pregnancy with offspring obesity and metabolic and vascular traits in childhood. *Circulation* 2010; **121**: 2557–2564.

40 Wolff S, Legarth J, Vangsgaard K, Toubro S, Astrup A. A randomized trial of the effects of dietary counselling on gestational weight gain and glucose metabolism in obese pregnant women. *Int J Obes (Lond)* 2008; **32** (3): 495–501.

41 Lovelady CA, Garner KE, Moreno KL, Williams JP. The effect of weight loss in overweight, lactating women on the growth of their infants. *N Engl J Med* 2000; **342** (7): 449–453.

42 Dodd JM, Turnbull D, McPhee AJ, Deussen AR, Grivell RM, Yelland LN, *et al.* Antenatal lifestyle advice for women who are overweight or obese: LIMIT randomised trial. *BMJ* 2014; **348**: 1–12.

43 Briley A, Barr S, Badger S, Bell R, Croker H, Godfrey KM, *et al.* A complex intervention to improve pregnancy outcome in obese women; the UPBEAT randomised controlled trial. *BMC Pregnancy Childbirth* 2014; **14**: 74.

44 Craigie AM, Macleod A, Barton KL, Treweek S, Anderson AS, on behalf of the WeighWell team. Supporting postpartum weight loss in women living in deprived communities: design implications for a randomised control trial. *Eur J Clin Nutr* 2011; **65**: 952–958.

45 Department of Health: Committee on Medical Aspects of Food Policy. *Dietary Reference Values of Food Energy and Nutrients for the United Kingdom: Report of the Panel on Dietary Reference Values of the Committee on (Reports of Health and Social Subjects: Volume 41)*. The Stationary Office: London, 1991.

CHAPTER 2

Nutrition and health in the early years

Judy More[1,2]

[1] School of Health Professions, Plymouth University, Plymouth, UK
[2] Child-nutrition.co.uk Ltd, London, UK

Introduction

Optimal nutrition supports growth, development and good health by providing adequate energy and nutrients. Other genetic and environmental factors that all interact to influence child development, growth and health in the pre-school age are as follows:
Individual influences
- Genotype
- Antenatal and prenatal environment and events
- Temperament
- Vision and hearing
Environmental influences
- Family, social and economic conditions
- Learning opportunities
- Parent child interaction
- Parenting behaviour
- Social network and community learning activities
- Public health programmes [1]

During the early years, feeding skills develop to ensure an increase in nutritional intake as energy and nutrient requirements increase with age. Breast milk provides adequate energy and nutrients for the first 4–6 months of life but thereafter complementary foods must be introduced alongside milk feeds to provide energy and nutrients in a more concentrated form. From 12 months onwards, energy and nutrient needs are provided by a varied and balanced diet based on five food groups (see Table 2.6) that each provides different nutrient profiles. The World Health Organization (WHO) sets energy and nutrient requirements for various age groups during infancy and childhood [2] but many countries have set their own national nutritional standards which may differ slightly from the WHO requirements.

Milk feeds for infants

Breast milk is the ideal milk for infants because it is both nutritionally adequate and contains a range of immunological substances that cannot be manufactured. Infant formula milk is the only substitute that is nutritionally adequate in the first 6 months

Early Years Nutrition and Healthy Weight, First Edition. Edited by Laura Stewart and Joyce Thompson.
© 2015 John Wiley & Sons, Ltd. Published 2015 by John Wiley & Sons, Ltd.

of life but it does not provide immunity. The benefits of breastfeeding include reduced risks of:

- gastrointestinal, urinary tract and respiratory infections
- otitis media (middle ear infection) until the age of 5–7 years
- both type 1 and type 2 diabetes mellitus
- constipation
- some childhood cancers (leukaemia and lymphomas, e.g. Hodgkin's disease)
- sudden infant death syndrome [3–6]

Evidence is controversial around whether breastfeeding reduces the following:

- risk of childhood obesity [7, 8]
- severity of the allergic conditions asthma and eczema [9, 10]

Breastfeeding is not an entirely instinctive process and low breastfeeding rates are often due to lack of support and advice for mothers to address common problems and difficulties. Influences on initiation and duration of breastfeeding include:

- The United Nations International Children's Emergency Fund (UNICEF) Baby Friendly status of the maternity unit where the baby is born. The UNICEF UK Baby Friendly Initiative provides a framework for the implementation of best practice for infant feeding in maternity units and is represented by the Ten Steps to Successful Breastfeeding [11].
- Direct skin-to-skin contact of infant with mother immediately after delivery until the first feeding is accomplished [12]. Putting the baby to the breast immediately after birth assists in developing the suckling reflex which is particularly strong for a short while after delivery.
- Extra support by trained professionals with special skills in breastfeeding to help with good positioning and technique [13].
- Peer support. Local peer support groups are particularly effective [14].
- Family support and encouragement.
- Supportive communities where breastfeeding is seen as the norm and facilities allow women to breastfeed on demand.

Reasons mothers cite for giving up breastfeeding earlier than would be ideal for their infant's health:

- Baby rejected breast
- Painful breasts/nipples
- Insufficient milk
- Took too long/tiring
- Mother or baby unwell
- Didn't like breastfeeding
- Baby could not be fed by others
- Returned to work or college [15]

Initiating, establishing and maintaining breastfeeding

Good positioning and attachment are essential for successful breastfeeding:

- Infants should be held so that:
  - they are close and facing the mother with their abdomen towards her
  - the baby's back, shoulders and neck are supported
  - they can easily tilt their head back
  - the head is in line with the body, nose to nipple, so that the neck is not twisted.
- The baby's mouth will gape, wide open in response to the rooting reflex to accept the nipple and it is important that the baby takes in the nipple and much of the areola. The lower lip should be turned out and the tongue under the mother's nipple.

The content of breast milk changes over time. Colostrum is produced in the first few days after birth, followed by transitional milk which is colostrum increasingly diluted with mature milk over the next 2 weeks and finally mature milk from about 3 weeks.

Over the first few days of life, infants feed infrequently and take minimal amounts of colostrum (21.5 ± 4.2 ml on day 1) [16]. A net loss in the baby's body weight which is mainly fluid is normal. Colostrum supply is under hormonal control and it is particularly high in proteins, especially immunoglobulins, which confer maternal immunity against infection. After about day three postpartum, the supply of transitional, and later mature, breast milk is determined largely by demand and is stimulated by regular, rather than prolonged, suckling. Mothers may need to feed every 2–3 hours or 8–12 times a day, but once lactation has become fully established, the time between feeds usually increases, although some infants continue to prefer smaller and more frequent feeds.

If the baby is unable to suckle from the breast, the mother can express her milk and feed by bottle, cup or spoon. Expressing 8–12 times a day will be necessary to establish a good milk supply and considerable practical and emotional support is important for these mothers.

Responsive feeding

Responsive feeding is feeding on demand beginning when the infant indicates hunger and allowing the infant to continue feeding until he/she ceases on becoming satiated. Responsive feeding thus allows the infant to regulate his/her energy intake. Younger infants feed more slowly, but as their sucking becomes more efficient with age, feeding takes less time.

The energy content of transitional and mature breast milk varies throughout a feed. At the beginning of the feed from each breast, the milk is low in fat and energy and higher in lactose and satisfies the infant's thirst, and as the feed progresses the fat and energy content increases satisfying the infant's hunger. Less milk (or none at all) may be taken from the second breast offered. At each feed, the first breast offered should be alternated so that both breasts receive equal stimulation and drainage.

Formula milk feeding

Up until 12 months of age, the only nutritionally adequate substitutes for breast milk are as follows:
1 Infant formula milk (suitable from birth)
2 Follow-on formula milk (can be used from 6 months *but is not necessary* as infant formula milk is suitable until 12 months of age)
The composition of these two types of milk must comply with government regulations.

Bottle-fed infants can be as responsively fed as breastfed babies. Daily intakes are approximately 150 ml/kg body weight/day after the first week, though this varies with each infant. The number of feeds per day and the volume taken at each feed will vary as in breastfeeding.

Holding bottle-feeding infants in a supportive, semi-upright position encourages eye contact and bonding with the caregiver. Angling the bottle so that the teat is always full of milk minimises the amount of air consumed.

The energy content of formula milks for infants is constant and higher than colostrum and transitional breast milk (see Table 2.1) and this may be a factor in the different growth patterns seen between breastfed and formula-fed infants [16, 17]. It is easier to overfeed a baby from a bottle by encouraging the infant to drink more even though they may have indicated they have had enough.

Table 2.1 Energy densities of breast milk and infant formula milk according to European regulations.

Breast milk per 100 g/100 ml			Infant formula milk
	Hester *et al.* [16]	Hosoi *et al.* [17]	European regulations
Colostrum	53.6 kcal (224 kJ)	57 kcal (238 kJ)	60–70 kcal (250–295 kJ)
Transitional milk	57.7 kcal (241 kJ)	63 kcal (263 kJ)	
Mature milk	65.2 kcal (273 kJ)	64 kcal (268 kJ)	

Additional fluids

No extra water is needed for exclusively breastfed infants even in very hot weather, as thirsty infants will simply demand more frequent feeds to obtain more fluid.

Formula-fed infants may become thirsty between feeds in very hot weather and additional drinks of cooled boiled water can be given so long as these do not interfere with the required intake of formula milk.

Fruit juices are not necessary as breast milk and infant formula milks contain sufficient vitamin C.

Complementary feeding

In addition to providing a more concentrated source of nutrition, complementary feeding alongside milk feeds provides the opportunity for infants to develop feeding skills and to learn to like a variety of new tastes and textures at an age when they are happy to do so. Continuing breastfeeding throughout complementary feeding affords maximum benefits for infants.

Age to begin complementary feed

In 2001, the WHO recommended exclusive breastfeeding until 6 months (26 weeks) of age [18] following a study in a developing country which reported that longer periods of exclusive breastfeeding protected against gastroenteritis [19]. This is a global population recommendation and the WHO advised that each infant should be considered individually. Some countries recommend weaning at about 6 months (e.g. UK, USA and Australia) while other countries recommend anytime between 4 and 6 months [20].

The following skills necessary for complementary feeding develop between 4 and 6 months of age [21]:

- Sitting with support with good head control to prevent choking
- An ability to move food from the front of the mouth to the back of the mouth to swallow

Further developmental stages that indicate readiness for complementary foods include:

- Putting toys and other objects in the mouth
- Chewing fists
- Watching others with interest when they are eating
- Seeming hungry between milk feeds or demanding feeds more often even though larger milk feeds have been offered

Night-time waking and crying are not necessarily signs of hunger at this age as infants of this age change their sleeping patterns and some are more easily aroused during periods of light sleep. There is no evidence that weaning onto solid food will help infants sleep through the night.

Table 2.2 Developmental stages of weaning.

Stage	Age guide	Skills to learn	New food textures to introduce
1	4–6 months	Taking food from a spoon Moving food from the front of the mouth to the back for swallowing Managing mashed food	Mashed foods
2	6–9 months	Moving lumps around the mouth Chewing lumps Self-feeding using hands and fingers Sipping from a cup	Mashed food with soft lumps Soft finger foods Liquids in a lidded beaker or cup
3	9–12 months	Chewing minced and chopped food Self-feeding attempts with a spoon	Hard finger foods Minced and chopped family foods

Table 2.3 Food groups and recommended servings for infants on three meals per day.

Food group	Foods included	Number of daily servings
Bread, other cereals and potatoes	Potatoes, yam, rice, couscous, pasta, millet, bread, toast chapatti, breakfast cereals, crackers, crispbread	3
Fruit and vegetables	Cooked or raw fruits and vegetables	3–4
Milk, cheese and yogurt	Yogurts, custard and other milk puddings, tofu	1–2
Meat, fish eggs, nuts and pulses	Meat, fish eggs, pulses, dhal, nut butters or finely ground nuts	1–2 (or 2–3 for vegetarians)
Fluid	Milk feeds Water with meals	On demand

Infants progress through the developmental stages of complementary feeding as they are given the opportunities to learn. Some progress faster than others, and Table 2.2 gives a rough guide.

Foods to offer

Offering one to two teaspoons of smooth mashed or pureed food at just one meal a day to begin allows the infant to learn how to manage food to the back of the mouth to swallow. The addition of solid foods to bottles of milk is not conducive to the infant learning new feeding skills and learning to accept new textures.

As the infant becomes adept, a second meal and then a third meal of different foods can be introduced. Once three meals are established, offering a variety of foods from the four main food groups will provide a range of nutrients to complement the milk. Offering finger foods at each meal in addition to spoon feeding allows the infant to develop self-feeding skills.

Table 2.3 shows the food groups and recommended number of daily servings. Meals should be nutrient dense and contain iron-rich foods. Foods high in fat and sugar do not have a place in the early weaning diet. WHO recommendations include the following:

• Salt and sugar should not be added to baby foods
• Honey should not be given before 12 months as there is a risk of botulism [22]

There is no evidence that delaying the introduction of any foods before 6 months reduces the incidence of allergy [23]. Recent evidence suggests that introducing gluten between 4 and 7 months while still breastfeeding may reduce the risk of coeliac disease and type 1 diabetes mellitus [20, 24].

Table 2.4 Pattern of feeding during weaning.

Stage	Age guide	Milk feeds	Meals	Variety of foods
1	4–6 months	5 down to 4	1–2	From one or two food groups
2	6–9 months	4 down to 3	3	Three different meals from four nutritious food groups One and two courses per meal Vitamin A & D supplements for breastfed babies
3	9–12 months	3 down to 2	3	Three different meals from four nutritious food groups Two courses per meal Vitamin A & D supplements for breastfed babies

Milk-based desserts can replace milk feeds at one and then two meals as the infant takes more food and two courses are offered at each meal time. The amount of breast milk or infant formula milk consumed by the infant will gradually reduce to about 500–600 ml/day towards the end of the first year. The pattern of feeding during complementary feeding is shown in Table 2.4.

Responsive feeding allows infants to regulate their energy intake by deciding how much solid food is eaten and how much milk is drunk. Infants who are happy to eat/drink more will:

- Open their mouth to accept a spoon of food or a nipple or bottle teat
- Pick up food and put it into their own mouth

When they have had enough they will:

- Keep their mouth shut when food is offered
- Turn their head away from food offered
- Put their hand in front of their mouth
- Push away a spoon, bowl or plate
- Hold foods in their mouth and refuse to swallow
- Spit out food repeatedly
- Cry, shout or scream
- Try to climb out of their high chair
- Gag or retch

Coercing an infant to eat or drink more than they wish or force feeding is counterproductive to developing a positive attitude to mealtimes and food.

The majority of infants are willing to try a wide variety of tastes and textures and they learn to like the foods they are offered [25]. The frequency with which they are offered a food, rather than the amount they eat, determines how quickly they learn to like a taste. By the end of their first year, infants should be eating family foods, and more the variety they have been offered by around 12 months, the wider the range of foods they will be familiar with and accept before food neophobia begins in their second year.

Homemade complementary foods give infants a wider experience of taste, texture and appearance than the uniformity found in factory-prepared commercial foods.

Additional fluids

Water can be offered from a cup or beaker with meals. It does not have to be boiled for babies over 6 months old, but freshly drawn tap water or bottled water from a clean cup can be given.

Sugary drinks, including fruit juices, cause dental caries especially when taken frequently from a bottle. In some countries, fruit juices are traditionally given to infants; however, this is not necessary as adequate vitamin C is provided from both:

- Breast milk or infant formula milk
- Fruits and vegetables included in meals

Tea and coffee are not suitable as they contain caffeine as well as tannins and polyphenols which inhibit iron absorption.

Recommended nutrient supplementation for infants

This varies from country to country. In those close to the equator, adequate vitamin D can be synthesised in the skin; however, this is less certain in countries of latitudes further from the equator.

In the UK, a supplement of vitamins A and D is recommended for:

- Breastfed infants from 6 months (or from 1 month if there is any doubt about the mother's nutritional status during pregnancy)
- Formula-fed infants over 6 months when they are taking less than 500 ml/day of formula [26, 27]

Infants at highest risk of vitamin D deficiency are those born to mothers who are themselves deficient in vitamin D. Mothers of Asian, African and Middle Eastern origin whose skin synthesis is limited either by living at latitudes further from the equator and or wearing concealing clothing, are most at risk. In areas of high incidence of vitamin D deficiency in the UK, vitamin D supplementation of infants is recommended from birth or within a few weeks.

Children 1–4 years of age

A combination of nutritious foods provides nutritional sufficiency except for vitamin D unless, as in some countries, commonly consumed foods are fortified with vitamin D. Most countries divide foods into groups of foods with similar nutrient profiles. These food groups are similar in different countries, although there is some variation in the naming of the food groups. They are shown in Table 2.5 with the recommended combination of daily servings.

Bread, rice, potatoes, pasta and other starchy foods

A mixture of some white and some wholegrain varieties can be offered as the fibre load from only wholegrain cereals may be too high for some pre-school-aged children. Excess fibre can trigger a feeling of satiety and reduce food intake thereby restricting energy and nutrient intake. Phytates in fibre reduce the absorption of certain nutrients and excess fibre may exacerbate loose stools in some toddlers.

Fruit and vegetables

Toddlers may be averse to the bitter taste of some vegetables or the challenging textures of some fruits and may eat a limited range of foods in this group. This should not be a cause for concern as this age is a time for learning to like fruits and vegetables and parents should encourage their toddlers to eat these foods by role modelling – eating with their toddlers and enjoying fruit and vegetables themselves.

Table 2.5 Food groups and recommended servings for children 1–4 years.

Food group	Foods included	Main nutrients supplied	Serving frequency
Bread, rice, potatoes, pasta and other starchy foods	Bread, chapatti, breakfast cereals, rice, couscous, pasta, millet, potatoes, yam, and foods made with flour such as pizza bases, buns, pancakes	Carbohydrate B vitamins Fibre Some iron, zinc and calcium	Serve at each meal and some snacks: five servings per day or four for vegetarians
Fruit and vegetable	Fresh, frozen, tinned and dried fruits and vegetables	Vitamin C Phytochemicals Fibre Carotenes	Offer at each meal and aim for three small servings of fruit and three small servings of vegetables
Milk, cheese and yogurt	Breast milk, formula milks, cow's milk, yogurts, cheese, calcium enriched soya milks, tofu	Calcium Protein Iodine Riboflavin	Three servings a day where one serving is 120 ml milk/ yogurt
Meat, fish, eggs nuts and pulses	Meat, fish eggs, pulses, dhal, nuts, seeds	Iron Protein Zinc Magnesium B vitamins Vitamin A Omega-3 long-chain fatty acids: eicospentaenoic acid and docosahexaenoic acid from oil-rich fish	Two servings a day or three for vegetarians Fish – twice per week including oil-rich fish once per week
Foods high in fat and/or sugar	Cream, butter, margarines, cooking and salad oils, mayonnaise, chocolate, confectionery, jam, syrup, crisps and other high-fat savoury snacks	Some foods provide: Vitamins D & E Omega-3 fatty acid: Alpha-linolenic acid	Very small servings to enhance flavour and enjoyment. In addition to but not instead of the other food groups
Fluid	Drinks	Water Fluoride in areas with fluoridated tap water	Six to eight drinks per day and more in hot weather or after extra physical activity

Milk, cheese and yogurt

After 12 months of age, milk intake should reduce to just three servings of milk, yogurt and cheese per day as this will meet calcium requirements. An excess of milk in the diet means less iron-rich foods are eaten and the risk of iron deficiency and anaemia increases [28, 29]. Whole (full-fat) milk provides more vitamin A than lower fat milks and is recommended as the milk drink for those 1–2 years in some countries. After 2 years of age, toddlers can change to semi-skimmed milk if they are eating well and growing normally but this is not necessary.

Meat, fish, eggs, nuts and pulses

Some toddlers find meat textures challenging and prefer soft tender cuts or meat products made from minced meat such as sausages, burgers and meatballs. When these foods are made from good-quality ingredients with a high lean meat and low salt content, they will make a valuable contribution to a healthy diet. Chicken, which often has a softer texture than red meat, is often preferred.

Offering fish twice a week including one portion as oily fish provides adequate omega-3 fats. Vegetarian children should combine pulses and nuts with foods from food group 1 (bread rice, potatoes, pasta and other starchy foods) to provide a source of first-class protein.

Foods high in fat and/or sugar

These high-energy foods add flavour and enjoyment to meals. Small amounts of them can be given in addition to the other food groups, but not instead of them. An excess of these foods will increase the likelihood of obesity. Some oil or fat high in omega-3 content should be included to provide the essential fatty acids.

Drinks

Six to eight drinks of about 100–120 ml can be offered throughout the day, with meals and snacks. More may be needed in very hot weather or after a lot of physical activity.

Water and milk are preferred drinks and can be given in a cup, beaker or glass. High-calorie, high-sugar drinks such as sugar-sweetened drinks, fruit juices and smoothies are not recommended. Drinks containing artificial sweeteners should be well diluted.

Bottles for milk or other drinks should be discontinued around 12 months as sucking on a bottle can be a comfort habit that is hard to break. Children who drink sweet drinks from bottles have a higher risk of dental caries [30].

Meal pattern

A regular meal pattern of three meals with two to three planned nutritious snacks per day is advised as pre-school-aged children may only take small quantities of food at any one time.

Two courses at each meal, a savoury course followed by a sweet course, ensure a wider variety of foods and nutrients will be offered. Parents/carers should be encouraged to think of the sweet course as a second opportunity to offer energy and nutrients and not offer it as a reward for finishing the savoury course.

Portion sizes

The appetite of under-5-year-olds varies from meal to meal and day to day and hence set portions sizes are not useful for them. The midpoints of the portion size ranges shown in Table 2.6 meet the UK and US recommendations for nutrients and average energy requirements for children aged 1–4 years when combined according to the specified number of daily servings [32]. They can be used to both reassure parents of young children who eat small amounts and to limit overeating particularly of food group 5 (foods high in fat and/or sugar).

Snacks

Planned nutrient-dense snacks can be made from combinations of foods from the first four food groups; examples are as follows:
- Fresh fruit (dried fruit can be cariogenic when eaten as a snack so it is not advised)
- Vegetable sticks, e.g. carrot, cucumber, pepper, baby corn and dips based on yogurt, low fat cream cheese or pulses such as hummus
- Wholegrain breakfast cereals with milk
- Cheese cubes and crackers or chapatti

Table 2.6 Portion size ranges for children aged 1–4 years.

Food group	Foods	Range of portion sizes
Bread, rice, potatoes, pasta	Bread	½–1 medium slice
and other starchy foods	Mashed potato	1–4 tbsp
Serve at each meal and some snacks	Pasta (cooked)	2–4 tbsp
5 servings per day or 4 for vegetarians	Rice	2–5 tbsp
Fruit and vegetables	Apple/pear/peach	¼–½ medium fruit
Serve at each meal and some snacks	Broccoli/cauliflower	1–4 small florets or ½–2 tbsp
3 servings of fruit and 3 servings	Clementine/tangerine/mandarin	½–1 fruit
of vegetables	Sweet corn	½–2 tbsp
Milk, cheese and yogurt	Cow's milk	100–120 ml or 3–4 fluid oz
3 servings per day	Grated cheese	2–4 tbsp
	Yogurt	1 average pot or 125 ml
Meat, fish, eggs, nuts and pulses	Baked beans in tomato sauce	2–4 tbsp
2 servings per day or 3 for vegetarians	Chicken drumsticks	½–1 drumstick
	Peanut butter	½–1 tbsp
	Scrambled egg	2–4 tbsp
	Tinned fish	½–1½ tbsp
Foods high in fat and sugar	Fruit crumble (e.g. apple	2–4 tbsp
Divided into four subgroups:	or rhubarb)	
1 serving per day of puddings, cake	Ice cream	2–3 heaped tbsp
or biscuits	Plain biscuits	1–2 biscuits
2 small servings per day of fats and oils	Honey/jam/syrup	1 tsp
1 serving per day of sauces and spreads	Butter/oil	Thinly spread or 1 tsp
1 serving per week of confectionery,	Tomato ketchup or gravy	1–2 tbsp
savoury snacks and sweet drinks	Crisps	4–6 crisps
	Sweets/confectionery	2–4 sweets

Reproduced with permission from Ref. 31. © Elsevier.
tbsp, tablespoon (15 ml); tsp, teaspoon (5 ml).

- Sandwiches, filled rolls and pitta breads
- French toast or toast with a range of spreads, used sparingly
- Slices of pizza with a plain dough base that has not been fried
- Yogurt and fromage frais
- Crumpets, scones, currant buns, teacakes, Scotch pancakes, fruit muffins and plain biscuits
- Homemade plain popcorn

Developmental changes in pre-school-aged children

How easily parents manage to feed their young children depends to some extent on parental knowledge and parenting skills. At the same time, developmental changes in toddlers affect how they respond to food and meals.

Neophobia

During their second year, toddlers develop a neophobic response to food becoming wary of trying new foods. This may be a survival mechanism to prevent mobile toddlers from poisoning themselves. This neophobic response usually peaks around 18 months and is more evident in some toddlers than others. If toddlers are being offered a wide variety of foods by around 12 months then they will enter their second year with a wider range of foods they recognise, like and readily accept [33].

Disgust and contamination fears

Children between 3 and 5 years may develop disgust fears and stop eating foods they may have previously enjoyed [34]. They will refuse a food on sight if it resembles something they find disgusting, for example they may find spaghetti suddenly looks like worms. Contamination fears occur around the same time and if a disliked food is put on a plate next to a liked food the toddler may refuse both foods.

Learning to like new foods

The neophobic response dissipates slowly [35, 36] in toddlers and young children if they are eating in social groups, as they learn by copying adults and other children that different foods are safe to eat. Family meals as frequently as possible ensure this and toddlers can be praised when they eat well. Some toddlers need to be offered a new food more than 10 times before they accept it as a liked food [31, 33].

Some toddlers have more problems than others [37] and there are two main reasons for this in healthy individuals:

1 Some become very rigid about the foods they will eat. They tend to be more emotional and more stubborn about what they will or will not do. They do not copy other children and do not copy other people's eating behaviour.
2 Others may be more sensory sensitive and have extreme reactions to touch, taste and smell. They may have problems with different textures of food and may have taken longer to progress from puree to lumpy food and onto more difficult textures. They may worry about getting their hands and face dirty and find it difficult to handle food and self-feed.

Exacerbating food refusal

Parental anxiety when toddlers eat selectively can exacerbate the problem, especially if parents try to coerce or force feed the child with food they are wary of or dislike. Up until 4–5 years of age, children's appetites are determined mainly by their energy and growth needs. They eat well at some times and less so at other times, and allowing them to decide the quantity they eat is the best strategy if weight gain is appropriate.

Some parents expect their toddlers to eat more than they need and coerce or force feed when the toddler is signalling they have had enough food. As meal times develop into a battle ground between toddler and parent, the toddler can lose their appetite just by becoming anxious as the meal time approaches. The signals toddlers use to indicate that they have had enough food include:

• Saying 'no'
• Keeping their mouth shut when food is offered
• Turning their head away from food being offered
• Pushing away a spoon, bowl or plate containing food
• Holding food in their mouth and refusing to swallow it
• Spitting food out repeatedly
• Crying, shouting or screaming
• Gagging or retching
• Trying to escape from the meal by climbing out of their chair or highchair

Common nutritional problems in pre-school-aged children

The common problems that arise from a poor diet include obesity, dental caries, iron deficiency anaemia, faltering growth and diarrhoea. Vitamin D deficiency and rickets occur in the absence of sufficient sunlight exposure and inadequate dietary vitamin D consumed either through supplements or fortified foods.

Impact of socio-economic status

The socio-economic status of families influences the food choices they are able to make. On very limited incomes, a family might prioritise the following over buying food:
- Rent/housing
- Heating and lighting
- Gas and electricity bills
- Clothes and shoes for children

Surveys of low-income families in the UK have found [38]:
- Almost half of parents had gone short of food, so the children had enough
- One in five families do not have enough money for food and have reduced or skipped meals
- Two in five families worried that food would run out before they had money to buy more
- Food insecurity was greatest in families with only one adult living with children.

Food accessibility is often poor in deprived areas:
- Foods available may be limited to a narrow range in small shops charging high prices
- Fruit and vegetables may be of poorer quality and if children do not eat them readily, parents may prefer to buy more filling foods that are cheaper but of lower nutritional value
- Accessible transport links to areas with larger markets and shops with competitively priced foods may be limited. Even with transport links to those shops, refrigeration and storage facilities within the home might restrict the better value bulk buys.

Welfare food schemes such as The Special Supplemental Nutrition Program for Women, Infants, and Children (WIC) in the USA and Healthy Start in the UK exist to make some nutritious foods affordable to low-income families. Not all eligible families take advantage of them for various reasons including lack of knowledge, poor accessibility and fear of being stigmatised [39, 40].

Parents may show their love to their children by treating them with relatively inexpensive sweet foods in place of unaffordable expensive toys and branded clothes and shoes that less-deprived children are given.

UK national nutritional surveys on under-5-year-olds have shown that:
- Poorer households have a less diverse diet and are less likely to experiment with new foods
- Although there is no significant difference in energy intake between different socio-economic groups, the intakes of most vitamins and minerals is lower in lower socio-economic groups
- Dental caries and iron deficiency anaemia are both more common in low-income households [30, 41].

Poor food choices may also be made by immigrants moving into areas where accessibility of their usual cultural foods is limited.

Putting the evidence into practice

A food diary for a child or a menu in a nursery can be assessed as in the example below to make sure foods consumed meet the criteria of nutritional adequacy. Menu or foods eaten in 1 day are listed in the left-hand column and each food or drink item is assigned to one or more food groups. Total servings in a day from each food group are assessed against recommendations:

All food and drinks consumed in 1 day	Food groups					Fluid
	Bread, rice, potato, pasta, other starchy food	Fruits and vegetables	Milk, cheese, yogurt	Meat, fish, eggs, nuts, pulses	Foods high in fat and/ or sugar	Drinks
Breakfast						
Breakfast cereal	1					
Milk on cereal			½			
Blueberries		1				
Water to drink						1
Mid-morning snack						
Banana slices		1				
Cup of milk to drink			1			1
Lunch						
Mini meatballs				1		
Pasta	1					
Cauliflower florets		1				
Apple crumble		1			1	
with ice cream					1	
Water to drink						1
Mid-afternoon snack						
Crackers with butter	1				1	
and cheese cubes			1			
Water to drink						1
Evening meal						
Fish and potato pie	1			1		
Carrot and cucumber sticks		1				
Plain yogurt mixed			1			
with strawberries		1				
Water to drink						1
Extra drinks of water						2
Totals	4	6	3½	2	3	7
Recommended	3–5 At each meal and some snacks	6 At each meal and some snacks	3	2–3	Some high fat foods	6–8 cups

This example can be seen to meet the average daily food group recommendations for 1–4-year-olds.

TAKE HOME MESSAGES

- Energy and nutrient requirements of infants from birth to about 6 months of age, can be satisfied by responsive feeding of breast milk or infant formula milk plus any nationally recommended supplements, for example vitamin D.
- The WHO recommends exclusive breastfeeding until 6 months of age to protect infants against gastroenteritis, but advises each infant should be considered individually.
- Nutritious complementary feeding from 4 to 6 months of increasingly complex textures encourages infants to develop their feeding skills, and to learn to like the taste and texture of the foods offered.
- Honey and foods with added sugar or salt should not be included in complementary feeding. Infants are born liking sweet tastes and need the opportunity to learn to like savoury tastes.
- Combining foods from five food groups plus any recommended supplements, for example vitamin D, satisfies the nutrient requirements of children aged 1–4 years.
- A balanced diet will not provide sufficient vitamin D if sunlight exposure is limited and foods are not fortified.
- Food neophobia is a normal developmental phase in toddlers and is seen more distinctly in some than in others.
- Inadequate nutrient intake is more common in pre-school-aged children in families within lower income populations.

References

1 Hopkins B, ed. *The Cambridge Encyclopaedia of Child Development.* Cambridge University Press: Cambridge, 2005.

2 World Health Organization. *Human Energy Requirements Report of a Joint FAO/WHO/UNU Expert Consultation,* Rome, Italy, 17–24 October 2001. Food and Agriculture Organization of the United Nations: Rome, 2004.

3 Quigley MA, Kelly YJ, Sacker A. Breastfeeding and hospitalisation for diarrhoeal and respiratory infection in the UK millennium cohort study. *Pediatrics* 2007; **119**: 837–842.

4 Quigley MA, Kelly YJ, Sacker A. Infant feeding, solid foods and hospitalisation in the first 8 months after birth. *Arch Dis Child* 2009; **941**: 48–50.

5 Ip S, Chung M, Raman G, *et al. Breastfeeding and Maternal and Infant Health Outcomes in Developed Countries. Evidence Report/Technology Assessment 153.* Agency for Healthcare Research and Quality: Rockville, 2007.

6 Horta BL, Bahl R, Martines JC, *et al. Evidence on the Long Term Effects of Breastfeeding: Systematic Reviews and Meta-Analyses.* World Health Organization: Geneva, 2007.

7 Jiang M, Foster EM. Duration of breastfeeding and childhood obesity: a generalised propensity score approach. *Health Serv Res* 2013; **48** (Pt 1): 628–651.

8 Hunsberger M. Early feeding practices and family structure: associations with overweight in children. *Proc Nutr Soc* 2014; **73** (1): 132–136.

9 Kramer MS, Kakuma R. Optimal duration of exclusive breastfeeding. *Cochrane Database Syst Rev* 2012; **8**: CD003517.

10 Al-Makoshi A, Al-Frayh A, Turner S, *et al.* Breastfeeding practice and its association with respiratory symptoms and atopic disease in 1-3-year-old children in the city of Riyadh, Central Saudi Arabia. *Breastfeed Med* 2013; **8** (1): 127–133.

11 Family and Reproductive Health: Division of Child Health and Development. *Evidence for the Ten Steps to Successful Breastfeeding.* World Health Organization: Geneva, 1998.

12 Mikiel-Kostyra K, Mazur J, Bołtruszko I. Effect of early skin-to-skin contact after delivery on duration of breastfeeding: a prospective cohort study. *Acta Paediatr* 2002; **91** (12): 1301–1306.

13 Renfrew MJ, McCormick FM, Wade A, *et al.* Support for healthy breastfeeding mothers with healthy term babies. *Cochrane Database Syst Rev* 2012; **5**: CD001141.

14 Chapman DJ, Morel K, Anderson AK, *et al.* Breastfeeding peer counselling: from efficacy through scale-up. *J Hum Lact* 2010; **26** (3): 314–326.

15 Bolling K, Grant C, Hamlyn B, *et al. Infant Feeding Survey 2005.* Information Centre: London, 2007.

16 Hester SN, Hustead DS, Mackey AD. Is the macronutrient intake of formula-fed infants greater than breast-fed infants in early infancy? *J Nutr Metab* 2012; **2012**: 1–13.

17 Hosoi S, Honma K, Daimatsu T, *et al.* Lower energy content of human milk than calculated using conversion factors. *Pediatr Int* 2005; **47**: 7–9.

18 Kramer MS, Kakuma R. *The Optimal Duration of Exclusive Breastfeeding: A Systematic Review.* World Health Organization: Geneva, 2001.

19 Kramer MS, Guo T, Platt RW, *et al.* Infant growth and health outcomes associated with 3 compared with 6 mo of exclusive breastfeeding. *Am J Clin Nutr* 2003; **78** (2): 291–295.

20 European Food Safety Authority (EFSA) Panel on Dietetic Products, Nutrition and Allergies (NDA). Scientific opinion on the appropriate age for introduction of complementary feeding of infants. *EFSA J* 2009; **7** (12): 1423–1461.

21 Carruth BR, Skinner JD. Feeding behaviours and other motor development in healthy children (2–24 months). *J Am Coll Nutr* 2002; **21** (2): 88–96.

22 World Health Organization. *Global Strategy for Infant and Young Child Feeding.* World Health Organization: Geneva, 2003.

23 Joneja JM. Infant food allergy: where are we now? *J Parenter Enteral Nutr* 2012; **36** (Suppl 1): 49–55.

24 Ivarsson A, Myléus A, Norström F, *et al.* Prevalence of childhood celiac disease and changes in infant feeding. *Pediatrics* 2013; **131** (3): 687–694.

25 Pliner P. The effects of mere exposure on liking for edible substances. *Appetite* 1982; **3**: 283–290.

26 National Institute for Health and Care Excellence. *Maternal and Child Nutrition: NICE Public Health Guidance 11.* NICE: London, 2008. http://www.nice.org.uk/nicemedia/live/11943/40097/40097.pdf (accessed on 7 April 2014).

27 Department of Health. *Weaning and the Weaning Diet. Report on Health and Social Subjects, no. 45.* HMSO: London, 1994.

28 Cowin I, Emond A, Emmett P, *et al.* Association between composition of the diet and haemoglobin and ferritin levels in 18-month-old children. *Eur J Clin Nutr* 2001; **55** (4): 278–286.

29 Thane CW, Walmsley CM, Bates CJ, *et al.* Risk factors for poor iron status in British toddlers: further analysis of data from the National Diet and Nutrition Survey of children aged 1.5–4.5 years. *Pub Health Nutr* 2000; **3** (4): 433–440.

30 Hinds K, Gregory JR. *National Diet and Nutrition Survey: Children Aged 1.5 to 4.5 Years. Volume 2. Report of the Dental Survey.* HMSO: London, 1995.

31 Birch L, Marlin DW. I don't like it, I never tried it: effects of exposure to food on two-year-old children's food preferences. *Appetite* 1982; **3**: 353–360.

32 More JA, Emmett PM. Evidenced-based, practical food portion sizes for preschool children and how they fit into a well balanced, nutritionally adequate diet. *J Hum Nutr Diet* 2014. doi:10.1111/jhn.12228.

33 Addessi E, Galloway AT, Visalberghi E, *et al.* Specific social influences on the acceptance of novel foods in 2-5-year-old children. *Appetite* 2000; **45**: 264–271.

34 Koivisto UK, Sjödén PO. Reasons for rejection of food items in Swedish families with children aged 2–17. *Appetite* 1996; **26**: 83–103.

35 Hill AJ. Developmental issues in attitudes to food and diet. *Proc Nutr Soc* 2002; **61**: 259–266.

36 Pliner P, Loewen ER. Temperament and food neophobia in children and their mothers. *Appetite* 1997; **28**: 239–254.

37 Wardle J, Cooke L. Genetic and environmental determinants of children's food preferences. *Br J Nutr* 2008; **99** (Suppl 1): 15–21.

38 Nelson M, Erens B, Bates B, *et al. Low Income Diet and Nutrition Survey.* The Stationary Office: London, 2007.

39 Department of Health. *Report on Health and Social Subjects No 51. Scientific Review of the Welfare Food Scheme.* The Stationary Office: London, 2002.

40 US Department of Agriculture. *Building a Healthy America: A Profile of the Supplemental Nutrition Assistance Program*, April 2012. http://www.fns.usda.gov/sites/default/files/BuildingHealthyAmerica.pdf (accessed 18 September 2014).

41 Gregory JR, Collins DL, Davies PSW, *et al. National Diet and Nutrition Survey: Children Aged 1½ and 4½ Years. Volume 1: Report of the Diet and Nutrition Survey.* HMSO: London, 1995.

Further reading

Healthy Child Programme e-Learning Programme. http://www.e-lfh.org.uk/projects/healthychild/index.html (accessed on 2 September 2014).

Infant and Toddler Forum Factsheets and Ten Steps for Healthy Toddlers. http://www.infantandtoddlerforum.org (accessed on 2 September 2014).

More J. *Infant, Child and Adolescent Nutrition: A Practical Handbook.* Boca Raton, FL: Taylor and Francis, 2013.

Morgan J, Dickerson JWT. *Nutrition in Early Life.* Chichester: John Wiley & Sons, Ltd, 2003.

Studies from the Avon Longitudinal Study of Pregnancy and Childhood. http://bristol.ac.uk/alspac (accessed on 2 September 2014).

UNICEF Baby Friendly Initiative. http://www.unicef.org.uk/babyfriendly (accessed on 2 September 2014).

CHAPTER 3

Defining and measuring childhood obesity

Charlotte M. Wright

Department of Child Health, School of Medicine, University of Glasgow, Glasgow, UK

Introduction

Obesity results from an energy imbalance, when more energy is consumed as food than is used by both activity and metabolic processes of the body. The human body has no way of excreting surplus energy, so any surplus energy is laid down in stores. Apart from quite modest amounts of glycogen in the liver, the main energy store of the body is adipose tissue (body fat). Our ability to lay down fat is crucial to health and longevity and it is what has allowed humans to survive long periods of famine and other adversities over the millennia. Thus, adipose tissue has an important and valued role in human metabolism and this is particularly the case in children. However, excess adipose tissue poses a long-term risk for health that has major public health significance in the modern age.

Variations in growth and adiposity with age

Young children rely even more heavily on fat stores than adults. Infants are born with only small fat stores and newborn infants, as well as growing rapidly in the first few weeks, lay down substantial stores which reach their peak at around the age of 1 year [1] (Figure 3.1). There are good evolutionary reasons for this. For the majority of human existence, it has been around this age that mothers become pregnant again and once a younger sibling is born, the infant will be weaned from the breast. Thus, in the first year, infants feed maximally and store any surplus as fat, to see them through the leaner years ahead. Whilst this is less critical today, infants are still growing at their fastest rate in the first year and also remain at high risk of infection, particularly if not breastfed. Thus, fat reserves are crucial to allow this rapid growth to continue.

After the first year, fat stores gradually diminish, whilst growth continues rapidly. Thus, the healthy infant or toddler tends to look plump in striking contrast to the lean appearance of the healthy pre-adolescent child (Figure 3.1). As puberty approaches, boys and girls show different changes in body composition (Table 3.1). For girls, the laying down of fat is an early and sustained feature of puberty whilst boys show much more rapid growth of muscle and lay down little fat, except sometimes immediately prior to the onset of the growth spurt (Figure 3.2).

Early Years Nutrition and Healthy Weight, First Edition. Edited by Laura Stewart and Joyce Thompson.
© 2015 John Wiley & Sons, Ltd. Published 2015 by John Wiley & Sons, Ltd.

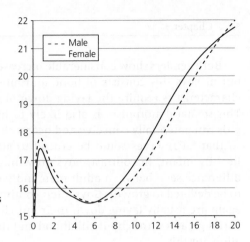

Figure 3.1 50th centile for BMI (UK 1990), genders compared. Reproduced with permission from WHO. © WHO.

Table 3.1 Advantages and disadvantages of different methods of assessing body composition in childhood.

Method	Advantages	Disadvantages
Waist circumference	Cheap portable and non-invasive	Hard to measure accurately in obese children; limited reference data. Associated with height as well as fat levels
Skinfolds	Relatively cheap, portable and fairly non-invasive; WHO norms available for pre-school-aged children	Training needed to measure accurately; limited reference data after age 5 years. Associated with height as well as fat levels
Bioelectrical impedance	Medium-cost equipment, non-invasive, relatively portable	Results require statistical manipulation before being interpretable. Only limited norms available for children. Imprecise compared to gold standard measures
Dual-energy X-ray absorptiometry (Dexa)	Non-invasive	Expensive, non-portable equipment. Imprecise compared to gold standard measures
Densitometry	Non-invasive; very accurate	Extremely expensive, non-portable equipment; requires skilled operation
Stable isotopes	Non-invasive; very accurate	Requires repeated urine collections, skilled operation and access to mass spectrometry. Very expensive

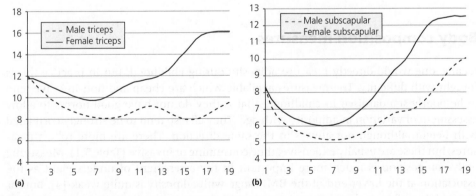

Figure 3.2 50th centile for (a) triceps and (b) subscapular skinfolds. Reproduced with permission from Ref. 2. © BMJ Publishing Group Ltd.

Both genders show considerable increase in body mass during puberty (Figure 3.1), but in boys this consists of bone and muscle, whilst in girls the secondary sexual characteristics require the laying down of considerable extra fat stores (Figure 3.2). This sexual dimorphism is also likely to have a strong evolutionary basis. Pubertal girls can potentially conceive and bear a child before the completion of their growth, so that fat reserves could be crucial to allow continued growth whilst gestating a healthy infant. In contrast, boys grow hugely in puberty, creating the large height difference seen between adult men and women, so that all energy consumed tends to be devoted to growth. Boys often continue to fill out after growth is completed but again are usually laying down their muscle and bony frame. Thus, natural adiposity varies greatly throughout childhood and the assessment of excess adiposity needs to allow for this.

How is adiposity measured in childhood?

As in adults, body mass index (BMI; weight Kg/height M^2) is the key measure. BMI does have some limitations that need to be properly understood, but these should not be overstated. The purpose of BMI is to assess a child's weight whilst allowing for the huge variation in height seen across childhood. Weight/height^2 largely adjusts for height at most ages in childhood, although at birth weight/height^3 is probably more effective [3]. It is important to be aware, however, that throughout childhood BMI is rarely completely independent of height. This is usually not of importance in clinical practice but is a main consideration for research and public health applications. BMI only measures total mass and much of the variation in BMI seen in healthy children is explained by variations in bony frame and muscle, as well as fat. However, at the top end of the BMI range, further increases in BMI tend to closely mirror increases in adiposity, rather than lean mass, which makes BMI very useful for assessing and monitoring obesity [4]. Obese children tend also to have higher muscle and possibly bone mass due to the extra load carried, particularly in the legs. However, this is a consequence of excess fat carried and for practical purposes is not important. Very athletic children may have higher BMI as a result of large muscle mass only, but this is only likely to be relevant within the normal range, for example in the boundary between healthy and overweight, rather than at high levels of BMI associated with obesity.

Body composition measures

Ideally, one would directly measure adiposity during childhood, but in practice this is fraught with difficulty. The measures available which are cheap and non-invasive tend to be poorly standardised in childhood, that is they do not have good norms to allow assessment of variation in adiposity with age. They all also tend to be strongly correlated with height, although not always in the same direction. There are more robust measures, but these are usually expensive, time consuming or invasive (Table 3.1). Measuring body composition is much more important in the assessment of underweight as the association at the lower end of the BMI range with adiposity is quite weak [4], but for overweight children, these measures are probably unnecessarily complex, particularly in a clinical setting.

How is obesity defined?

BMI is therefore the measure of choice for assessing childhood obesity. While standards exist from birth, BMI is generally not recommended as a measure before the age of 2 years due to the difficulty in obtaining a robust estimate of length before that age [5]. As BMI varies so much with age, it cannot be used as a raw measure, but must be compared to a standard or reference before it can be interpreted. Until recently, all growth charts for weight and height as well as BMI were reference standards, which simply described the normal distribution of measurements within the population of interest. However, recently there has been recognition that the distribution of a measurement seen in the population may not always be the healthy distribution and this particularly applies to BMI. Thus, the question of which norm a child's BMI should be compared to is crucial. For obesity, the problem is that a contemporary growth reference will not describe the healthy pattern of growth as it will also include many unhealthy obese children. Thus, norms derived from modern children would define a much wider range of children as being 'normal', and this is unhelpful in public health terms.

For pre-school-aged children, the solution is to use the World Health Organization (WHO) growth standard. This was derived from six separate populations around the world sampled between 1997 and 2003 who were all breastfed for the first year of life, exclusively for at least 4 months and living in healthy circumstances [6]. This standard has been widely adopted and has been implemented in the UK for children aged up to age 4 since 2009–2010. Beyond that age in the UK, the pragmatic solution to this problem has been to continue using the UK 1990 growth reference, and these two sources are joined on the new UK growth charts at age 4 years and termed the UK–WHO reference [5]. The UK 1990 presents reference data for BMI from children measured in the 1980s [7], presumptively before the obesity epidemic had fully gathered pace. It is of note that the centiles for both weight and BMI from the first year onwards on the WHO standard are nearly 1 centile space lower than for the UK 1990 [8], even though the UK 1990 are based on children growing up 25 years ago (Figure 3.3). This suggests that even in the 1980s, children were perhaps already on average above the optimum weight.

Elsewhere in the world, the WHO 2007 reference is available for use in school-age children. This does not have the validity of the pre-school age standard, since it is based solely on data from children in the USA collected in the 1970s [9], but it gives similar results to UK 1990 except later in the teens when it has higher upper thresholds. In the USA, the Center for Disease Control (CDC) BMI references are used. These are based on more recently collected US data and it is of note that their upper centiles are much the highest (Figure 3.3).

What thresholds should be used?

We then have to decide what centile within a particular growth reference or standard should be used to define obesity. Many different thresholds are used and this can cause great confusion. These are summarised in Tables 3.2 and 3.3. In the USA the 85th centile is used to define overweight and the 95th centile is used to define obesity for both population surveillance (epidemiological) and clinical use. In the UK, lower thresholds such as the 85th and 95th centiles are used for epidemiological purposes to give an overview of the whole population at risk of overweight [10]. This has the advantage of being

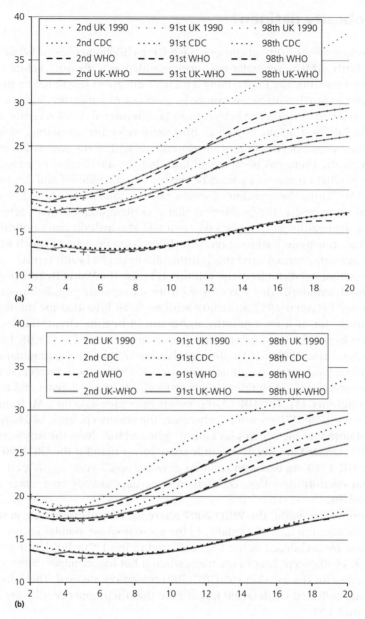

Figure 3.3 BMI compared to WHO, UK 1990 and CDC references in (a) girls and (b) boys.

Table 3.2 BMI thresholds in use in UK and USA.

US threshold	Centile
Underweight	5
Overweight	85
Obese	95

Table 3.3 BMI thresholds in use in UK and USA.

UK threshold	Centile
Thin (clinical)	0.4
Low BMI (epidemiological)	2
At high risk of overweight (epidemiological)	85
Overweight (clinical)	91
At high risk of obesity (epidemiological)	95
Clinical obesity (clinical)	98
Severe obesity (clinical)	99.6
Morbid obesity	3–3.5 SD

inclusive and not missing out children who are carrying excess body fat (overfat), as well as supplying sufficient numbers to generate stable statistics for reporting purposes. However, it must be recognised that such thresholds lack specificity and will include many children who are not overfat at all as well as others who will revert to a healthy weight at later ages. More extreme thresholds are therefore more helpful for clinical purposes and the higher the threshold the more likely it is that most or all children so classified are both currently overfat and at risk of future obesity. It is children in these upper categories who have an undeniable increased risk both of adulthood obesity and premature mortality [11, 12]. It is also of note that it is these children who are most recognisably overweight, even to their parents [13].

As these are thresholds based on less-obese populations, the proportion above each will usually be much higher than the expected value implied by the centile. Thus, for example, in England 10–20% of children are above the 95th centile (depending on age) where 5% would be expected [14]. This problem is avoided by an entirely different option, the International Obesity Task Force (IOTF) thresholds. These simply classify children into 'healthy', 'overweight' and 'obese' using a merged international dataset with thresholds in childhood set to correspond with BMIs of 25 and 30 at age 18 years [15]. The overweight threshold approximates to the UK 1990 91st centile while the obese threshold is somewhere between the 98th and 99.6th centiles. This is the most useful approach to use for international epidemiological comparisons, but this has limited use for clinical purposes as there are only two upper categories, which do not allow assessment of change within a category and the obese category is quite stringent.

What chart tools are available to assess overweight?

The new UK growth charts all now include a BMI centile lookup (Figure 3.4) which, once the weight and height have been plotted, allows you to use the centiles to read off the BMI centile, accurate to within a quarter of a centile space. On the school age charts, there is also a BMI centile grid at the top of the growth chart where this centile can be plotted, so that the BMI centile can be monitored over time. This is very useful for initial screening but is not suitable for the assessment of very obese children as there are no centile lines above 99.6th centile. Many full BMI charts have similar limitations. For example, the CDC charts and their electronic calculators (http://apps.nccd.cdc.gov/dnpabmi/) provide no information beyond whether a child's BMI is above the 95th centile. The new Royal College of Paediatrics and Child Health (RCPCH) UK BMI charts, published both as individual charts and as part of the new Childhood and Puberty Close Monitoring Chart, now show 'high lines' above the

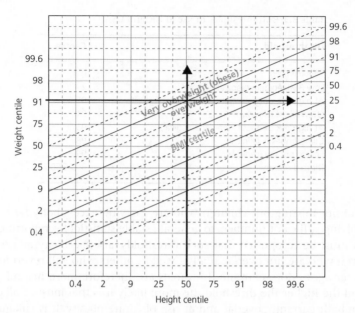

Figure 3.4 BMI lookup as provided on UK-WHO 2–18 years growth chart. Draw a vertical line from height centile on *X*-axis to meet a horizontal line drawn from the weight centile on the *Y*-axis. Where the two lines cross, read off BMI centile from the diagonal lines: 98th centile in this example. Reproduced with permission from Royal College of Paediatrics and Child Health, UK. © Royal College of Paediatrics and Child Health, UK.

99.6th centiles at 3.33, 3.66 and 4 standard deviations (SD) (Figure 3.5). These charts can all be viewed on http://www.RCPCH.ac.uk/growthcharts and purchased from Harlow Printing Limited, Maxwell Street, South Shields, Tyne and Weir, NE33 4PU, UK. In the USA, one unit has described creating a new chart with additional high lines, defined by the extent to which the BMI is above the 95th centile, expressed as a percentage of the 95th centile for that age and gender [16] but these are not yet generally available.

Putting the evidence into practice

A school nurse is asked to see the concerned parent of 15-year-old girl Chelsea, whose General Practitioner (GP) has suggested that she should lose weight, when she presented with stretch marks. The GP told them that Chelsea was above the clinically obese thresholds and gave general advice about diet and exercise. Mum is keen to help and went on the web and downloaded a US BMI chart to use to monitor progress. She is puzzled to find on this chart that Chelsea is only classified as overweight. She remarks that she knows her daughter has 'filled out a bit' recently but that when she was younger she was worried that she might be underweight. The school nurse has previous heights and weights which show she had tracked the 50th centile until puberty but has risen sharply in the last few years. The school nurse explains that it is normal and healthy to look slim in the pre-adolescent years, and that while it is also normal to put on weight as you go into puberty, Chelsea has gained weight faster than is considered healthy. She explains that the thresholds for overweight in USA are higher than in the UK, as they are based on a more overweight population.

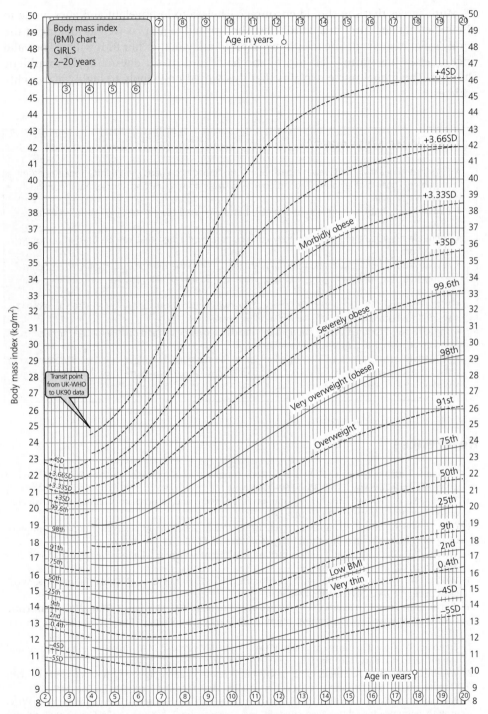

Figure 3.5 BMI chart as provided on UK-WHO 2–18 years growth chart. Reproduced with permission from Royal College of Paediatrics and Child Health, UK. © Royal College of Paediatrics and Child Health, UK.

Mum agrees that she should encourage Chelsea to lose weight and goes home to discuss letting her enrol in a dance class she wanted to join, as well as looking at the family's diet in general. She telephones later to ask whether her BMI will still be valid once Chelsea has started dancing, as she has heard that it doesn't apply to athletic children. The school nurse explains that this would only apply to highly active elite athletes!

TAKE HOME MESSAGES

- Fat stores in healthy infants reach a peak at around the age of 1 year, then decline until the onset of puberty, when girls lay down fat and boys tend to lay down bone and muscle, both resulting in a steady rise in BMI.
- BMI measures both fat and lean body mass, but a high BMI corresponds closely to high fatness levels.
- There are no reliable measures of body composition for children that can be used in a routine clinical setting.
- A wide range of BMI charts and thresholds are used, but in the UK, the 95th centile is most commonly used for epidemiological purposes, while the 91st and 98th centiles are used in clinical practice.
- In the USA, the 85th centile defines 'at risk of overweight' and 95th centile defines 'at risk of overweight' for both epidemiological and clinical purposes.
- The IOTF classification provides standard thresholds for overweight and obesity for use for research and epidemiological comparisons worldwide.
- UK growth charts provide a BMI centile lookup on the standard charts and a detailed BMI chart on the Childhood and Puberty Close Monitoring Chart, which allow assessment of children with BMI well above the healthy range.

References

1 Fomon S, Haschke F, Ziegler E, Nelson S. Body composition of reference children from birth to age 10 years. *Am J Clin Nutr* 1982; **35**: 1169–1175.
2 Tanner JM, Whitehouse RH. Revised standards for triceps and subscapular skinfolds in British children. *Arch Dis Child* 1975; **50** (2): 142–145.
3 Cole TJ. Weight/height p compared to weight/height 2 for assessing adiposity in childhood: influence of age and bone age on p during puberty. *Ann Hum Biol* 1986; **13** (5): 433–451.
4 Wright CM, Garcia AL. Child undernutrition in affluent societies: what are we talking about? *Proc Nutr Soc* 2012; **71** (4): 545–555.
5 Wright CM, Williams AF, Elliman D, Bedford H, Birks E, Butler G, *et al.* Using the new UK-WHO growth charts. *BMJ* 2010; **340**: 647–650.
6 de Onis M, Garza C, Victora CG, Onyango AW, Frongillo EA, Martines J. The WHO Multicentre Growth Reference Study: planning, study design, and methodology. *Food Nutr Bull* 2004; **25** (1): 15–26.
7 Freeman JV, Cole TJ, Chinn S, Jones PRM, White EM, Preece MA. Cross sectional stature and weight reference curves for the UK, 1990. *Arch Dis Child* 1995; **73**: 17–24.
8 Wright C, Lakshman R, Emmett P, Ong KK. Implications of adopting the WHO 2006 Child Growth Standard in the UK: two prospective cohort studies. *Arch Dis Child* 2008; **93** (7): 566–569.
9 de Onis M, Onyango AW, Borghi E, Siyam A, Nishida C, Siekmann J. Development of a WHO growth reference for school-aged children and adolescents. *Bull World Health Organ* 2007; **85** (9): 660–667.
10 Scientific Advisory Committee on Nutrition (SACN)/Royal College of Paediatrics and Child Health (RCPCH). *Consideration of issues around the use of BMI centile thresholds for defining underweight, overweight and obesity in children aged 2–18 years in the UK*, 2007. http://www.sacn.gov.uk/pdfs/sacnrcpch_position_statement_bmi_thresholds.pdf (accessed 6 April 2014).

11 Hoffmans M, Kromhout D, de Lezenne Coulander C. The impact of body mass index of 78,612 18-year old Dutch men on 32 year mortality from all causes. *J Clin Epidemiol* 1988; **41** (8): 749–756.

12 Allebeck P, Bergh C. Height, body mass index and mortality: do social factors explain the association. *Public Health* 1992; **106**: 375–382.

13 Parkinson KN, Drewett RF, Jones AR, Dale A, Pearce MS, Wright CM, *et al.* When do mothers think their child is overweight? *Int J Obes* 2011; **35** (4): 510–516.

14 Lifestyle Statistics Team/Health and Social Care Information Centre. *National Child Measurement Programme: England, 2012/13 School Year*. London: Health and Social Care Information Centre, UK Government Statistical Service, 11 December 2013. http://www.hscic.gov.uk/catalogue/PUB13115/nati-chil-meas-prog-eng-2012-2013-rep.pdf (accessed 10 September 2014).

15 Cole T, Bellizzi M, Flegal K, Dietz W. Establishing a standard definition for child overweight and obesity worldwide: international survey. *BMJ* 2000; **320** (6): 1240–1243.

16 Gulati AK, Kaplan DW, Daniels SR. Clinical tracking of severely obese children: a new growth chart. *Pediatrics* 2012; **130** (6): 1136–1140.

CHAPTER 4
Early life risk factors for childhood obesity

John J. Reilly and Adrienne R. Hughes

Physical Activity for Health Group, School of Psychological Sciences & Health, University of Strathclyde, Glasgow, UK

Established early life risk factors for childhood obesity

A number of early life risk factors for obesity have been identified and summarised in systematic reviews of mainly observational studies [1–4]. These risk factors either promote excessive energy intake or promote inadequate energy expenditure, or both.

Early life risk factors for obesity at age 7 years identified by ALSPAC study

In the large Avon Longitudinal Study of Parents and Children (ALSPAC) in England, 25 potential infant and early childhood risk factors were tested to see if they were actually associated with obesity at age 7 years: eight risk factors were associated with later obesity risk [5]. The effect of each risk factor for obesity by age 7 years is described in the following text and is summarised in Table 4.1.

Rapid early growth

Growing rapidly early in infancy and early childhood is a predictor of increased risk of later obesity which has been identified by many studies including ALSPAC [5] and confirmed by systematic reviews [1–4]. The reasons why rapid early growth is associated with later obesity are not completely clear at the moment, but animal studies confirm that there are biological mechanisms (as well as environmental and behavioural mechanisms) which lead from rapid early growth to later obesity, and in humans rapid early growth increases the risk of later obesity substantially.

Adiposity rebound is the period in early childhood where body mass index (BMI) begins to increase from a nadir and normally occurs between age 5 and 7 years [6]. In the ALSPAC study [5], early adiposity rebound (younger age at onset) had the strongest association with later obesity, much stronger than any of the other risk factors identified

---

Early Years Nutrition and Healthy Weight, First Edition. Edited by Laura Stewart and Joyce Thompson.
© 2015 John Wiley & Sons, Ltd. Published 2015 by John Wiley & Sons, Ltd.

Table 4.1 Well-established early life risk factors for childhood obesity in ALSPAC [5].

Risk factors	Magnitude of risk for obesity at 7 years
Early rapid growth	
Very early adiposity rebound (before age 3.5 years)	AOR 15 vs. later adiposity rebound (after age 5 years)
Every 100 g increase in birth weight	5% increase in risk (AOR 1.05/100 g increase)
Every 100 g increase in weight from 0 to 12 months	6% increase in risk (AOR 1.06/100 g increase)
Catch-up growth (weight gain of >0.67 standard deviation scores in first 2 years)	AOR 2.6 vs. no catchup
Parental obesity (both parents obese)	AOR 10 vs. neither parent obese
>8 hours/week of TV viewing at age 3 years	AOR 1.55 vs. <4 hours/week
<10.5 hours/night of sleep at age 3 years	AOR 1.45 vs. ≥12 hours/night of sleep

AOR, adjusted odds ratio. Formula feeding was not identified as a risk factor in ALSPAC; however, meta-analyses [3, 4] have reported a 15–30% reduction in risk with breastfeeding.

including parental obesity. The adjusted odds ratio (AOR)[1] for obesity at age 7 years was *15* for children with 'very early adiposity rebound' (before age 3.5 years) compared to those with later adiposity rebound (after age 5 years), while the AOR for obesity at age 7 years was *10* for those with two obese parents (compared to those with both parents non-obese). Early adiposity rebound reflects a period of rapid and excessive weight gain in early childhood, and other studies [6, 7] have confirmed that early adiposity rebound predicts substantially increased risk of later obesity.

In the same ALSPAC study, rapid early growth at other times in early life, and expressed in other ways, was also related to later risk of obesity (Table 4.1), though not so strongly, as timing of adiposity rebound. These included 'catch-up' growth (the AOR for obesity at age 7 was *2.6* for those who gained >0.67 of a standard deviation score in weight between birth and age 2 years versus those with no catch-up growth in the first 2 years), higher weight gain from birth to 12 months (6% increase in risk of obesity at 7 years for every additional 100 g gain in weight in first year) and having a relatively high body weight at various points in early life including a higher birth weight (a 5% increase in risk of obesity at 7 years for every additional 100 g in birth weight).

In summary, rapid early growth, and high body weight, whether in infancy or in early childhood, both confer substantially increased risk of obesity. One logical conclusion of this evidence is that we could prevent obesity directly, by growth modifying interventions in early life. Such interventions have in fact been quite scarce so far and have been hindered by concerns over possible adverse effects of growth modification. One notable exception, where growth modification via reduced protein intake in infant formula was the intervention, is the European Childhood Obesity Trial (ECOT) [8]. Early results from the ECOT suggest that reducing the protein content of infant formula is a safe way of modifying the growth of formula-fed babies, and it would appear to reduce their risk of later obesity [8]. The other early life risk factors for later obesity discussed in the following

---

[1]An odds ratio (OR) is a measure of association between an exposure (e.g. parental obesity) and an outcome (e.g. child obese at age 7 years). In this example, the OR represents the odds that an outcome will occur given a particular exposure (e.g. having two obese parents), compared to the odds of the outcome occurring in the absence of that exposure (e.g. neither parent obese). The OR ratio can be used to determine whether a particular exposure is a risk factor for a particular outcome, and to compare the magnitude of various risk factors for that outcome. An adjusted odds ratio (AOR) controls for other variables (e.g. material education and gender) that may also influence the outcome and exposure.

may operate in part by promoting rapid early growth, and so modifying them may help prevent obesity via a reduction in rapid early growth.

Formula milk feeding in infancy

Formula milk feeding was not identified as a risk factor in the ALSPAC study; however, a substantial body of evidence from observational studies suggests that formula feeding is a risk factor for later obesity [1, 3, 4, 9]. A recent meta-analysis [3] reported a 15% decrease in the risk of later obesity among children who were 'ever breastfed' in the first year of life (including exclusively breastfed, ever breastfed or fed a mixture of formula milk and breast milk) compared with children who were exclusively formula-fed. Another meta-analysis found that mothers who breastfed exclusively for 4–6 months, as widely recommended, reduced their infant's risk of later obesity by around 30% compared to the risk for infants who were formula fed [4].

There is still some controversy over whether or not formula feeding actually causes later obesity, and there are probably several mechanisms, not yet understood fully, which operate to reduce the risk of obesity in breastfed babies. The act of bottle feeding may lead the baby to passivity in feeding, increasing the risk of passive overconsumption (which may lead to rapid early growth), and in one study even breast milk was overconsumed when fed via a bottle [10]. Even if there is doubt about the benefits of breastfeeding for obesity prevention, there are no serious doubts about the benefits of breastfeeding for mothers and their babies, and so health professionals and policy makers should not be concerned about promoting greater breastfeeding initiation and more exclusive breastfeeding for longer periods. Recently, several research-based obesity prevention interventions [11–13] have promoted breastfeeding and other appropriate feeding practices in infancy (e.g. introducing solids foods at 6 months), using response-feeding practices, including the 'Healthy Beginnings' study [12], which reported positive intervention effects on BMI at age 2 years.

Television viewing

Most of the studies in early life on relationships between sedentary behaviour and risk of later obesity have focused on television (TV) viewing. While TV viewing is only one form of sedentary behaviour, it is one which is particularly available to infants and young children: in older children and adolescents, other forms of screen-based sedentary behaviour are more available via their increasingly easy access to a wider range of other media. Exposure to TV viewing is fairly common in infants and young children, and it probably 'tracks' with age, that is those infants and young children with highest exposure to TV in early life tend to also have the highest exposure to TV later in life [14].

In the ALSPAC study [5], TV viewing in children at age 3 years was reported by their parents, and this was strongly predictive of risk of obesity at age 7 years, with risk increasing as TV exposure increased. Compared to those reported to watch less than 4 hours of TV per week at age 3 years, obesity risk was 37% higher for those reported to watch 4–8 hours/week and 55% for those reported to watch more than 8 hours/week (Table 4.1).

As with most of the other early life risk factors for later obesity, the mechanisms which link TV viewing to obesity are not fully understood, but TV exposure probably promotes both a reduction in energy expenditure and an increase in energy intake. Watching TV in pre-school-aged children is associated with excessive energy intake [15] and TV viewing (e.g. during mealtimes) may encourage a passive overconsumption of energy: internal cues indicating satiety may be overridden by the distraction of TV [16]. Since TV viewing in early life has been consistently and strongly linked to later obesity risk, and since reductions in TV viewing would probably benefit child health and development in other ways, reducing TV viewing is a common feature in many of the research-based interventions aimed at preventing obesity in early life [17, 18]. In the recent US 'Healthy Kids Happy Homes' study [17], for example, an important element in the intervention is to promote an increase in families eating together with a reduction in eating meals in front of the TV. Evidence-based guidelines [19] recommend limiting TV viewing and other screen-based behaviours (e.g. computer, electronic games) to 1 hour/day or less for children aged 2–4 years, and screen time is not recommended for children under 2 years.

Lack of sleep/disrupted sleep

A number of studies have now shown fairly consistently that reduced sleep and/or disrupted sleep in infancy and early childhood promote an increased risk of later obesity, and these studies have been summarised in recent systematic reviews and meta-analyses [1]. In the ALSPAC study, those children with less than 10.5 hours sleep per night at age 3 years had a 45% increase in risk of obesity at age 7 compared to those with more than 12 hours sleep per night.

Staying awake longer may increase risk of obesity in part by the simple action of increasing exposure to the modern obesity-promoting environment, but other mechanisms probably contribute, and lack of sleep impairs appetite regulation and promotes overconsumption by hormonal mechanisms. A secular trend to reduced sleep duration in children may have contributed to the obesity epidemic, and increasing sleep duration is likely to have a wide range of benefits for child health and development [20]. As a result, promotion of sleep (e.g. sleep routines, removing TV screens from bedrooms) has been featuring increasingly in early life–based research interventions aimed at preventing childhood obesity. In the 'Healthy Kids Happy Homes' intervention, for example, the promotion of a sleep routine is an integral part of the intervention [17].

Early life risk factors for later obesity not studied in ALSPAC

Low physical activity and sugar-sweetened drink consumption in early childhood were not studied in ALSPAC; however, systematic reviews have generally supported the view that these behaviours increase the risk of later obesity [1, 21]. Recent systematic reviews found that a daily physical activity of less than 30 minutes and consumption of sugar-sweetened drinks in early life (0–5 years) were associated with later overweight and obesity [1]. However, it is difficult to estimate the size of the obesity risk associated with these behaviours due to differences in the populations studied and in the methods used to measure, for example physical activity. Several of the research-based obesity prevention interventions aimed at infants and young children include a focus on encouraging physical activity and consumption of water and milk [11–13, 17, 18]. Recommended levels of physical activity and the impact of physical activity in early life are discussed in Chapter 5. It is also important to note that maternal factors (i.e. smoking, weight gain and diabetes during pregnancy) and socio-economic status are strongly related to later obesity risk [1, 3, 5]; the impact of maternal weight gain and socio-economic status are discussed in Chapter 1.

Putting the evidence on early life risk factors for childhood obesity into practice

Knowledge of the well-established modifiable risk factors in early life for childhood obesity should make it possible for health professionals, early years workers, child care providers and families to direct their efforts towards changing these 'obesogenic' behaviours (i.e. formula milk feeding, screen time, lack of sleep, low physical activity and sugar-sweetened drinks). Table 4.1 describes the size of the risk associated with each of these behaviours. Modifying these behaviours in infancy and early childhood may help to reduce the risk of obesity in later childhood, possibly by reducing rapid early growth so that children are on a healthier weight trajectory in the long term and will benefit child health and development in other ways. Recommendations on infant feeding, diet, physical activity and sedentary behaviour are available and are discussed in other chapters, along with guidance on *how* to change these behaviours (e.g. using behavioural change techniques).

Knowledge of the main behavioural risk factors can also help health professionals identify infants and young children who are at high risk of developing obesity, and so directing efforts and limited resources at high risk individuals if that is desirable. Frequent monitoring of growth in infancy and early childhood would identify individuals who are growing rapidly. In the ALSPAC study [5], very early adiposity rebound (before age 3.5 years) had the strongest association with obesity risk at age 7 years. Identifying timing of adiposity rebound is feasible in clinical practice and involves plotting three to four BMI measurements on a standard BMI for age chart between the ages of 2.5–5 years. Other indices of rapid growth (e.g. catch-up growth, defined as a gain in weight standard deviation score of >0.67 between birth and age 2 years) could also be used to identify infants and toddlers at higher risk of later obesity.

TAKE HOME MESSAGES

- Established early life risk factors for childhood obesity include rapid early growth, formula milk feeding, screen time, lack of sleep, low physical activity and sugar-sweetened drinks.
- Early adiposity rebound (before age 3.5 years) had the strongest association with obesity risk at age 7 years in ALSPAC.
- Modifying these risk factors in infancy and early childhood may reduce the risk of obesity in later childhood and will benefit child health and development in other ways.
- Frequent monitoring of growth in infancy and early childhood would identify individuals who are growing rapidly and are therefore at high risk of developing obesity in later childhood.

References

1 Monasta L, Batty GD, Cattaneo A, Lutje V, Ronfani L, van Lenthe FJ, Brug J. Early-life determinants of overweight and obesity: a review of systematic reviews. *Obes Rev* 2010; **11**: 695–708.
2 Baird J, Fisher D, Lucas P, Kleijnen J, Roberts H, Law, C. Being big or growing fast: systematic review of size and growth in infancy and later obesity. *BMJ* 2005; **331**: 929–935.
3 Weng SF, Redsell SA, Swift JA, Yang M, Glazebrook CP. Systematic review and meta-analyses of risk factors for childhood overweight identifiable during infancy. *Arch Dis Child* 2012; **97**: 1019–1026.
4 Horta BL, Bahl R, Martines JC, Victora CG. Evidence on the long-term effects of breastfeeding. *WHO Library* 2007.
5 Reilly JJ, Armstrong J, Sherriff A, Dorosty AR, Emmett PM, Ness AR, *et al*. Early life risk factors for obesity in contemporary children: cohort study. *BMJ* 2005; **330**: 1357–1362.
6 Taylor RW, Grant AM, Goulding A, Williams S. Early adiposity rebound: a review of papers linking this to subsequent obesity in children and adults. *Curr Opin Clin Nutr Metab Care* 2005; **8**: 607–611.
7 Rolland-Cachera MF, Deheeger M, Maillot M, Bellisle F. Early adiposity rebound: causes and consequences for obesity in children and adults. *Int J Obes* 2006; **30**: s11–s17.
8 Koletzko B, von Kries R, Closa R, Escribano J, Scaglioni S, Giovannini M, *et al*. Lower protein in infant formula is associated with lower weight up to age 2 years: a randomized clinical trial. *Am J Clin Nutr* 2009; **89**: 1836–1845.
9 Ip S, Chung M, Raman G, Chew P, Magula N, Devine D, *et al*. Breastfeeding and maternal and infant health outcomes in developed countries. *Evid Rep Technol Assess* 2007; **153**: 1–186.
10 Li R, Fein SB, Grummer-Strawn LM. Do infants fed from bottles lack self-regulation of milk intake compared with directly breastfed infants? *Pediatrics* 2010; **125**: e1386.
11 Daniels LA, Mallan KM, Battistutta D, Nicholson JM, Perry R, Magarey A. Evaluation of an intervention to promote protective infant feeding practices to prevent childhood obesity: outcomes of the NOURISH RCT. *Int J Obes* 2012; **36**: 1292–1298.
12 Wen LM, Baur LA, Simpson JM, Rissel C, Wardle K, Flood VM. Effectiveness of home based early intervention on children's BMI at age 2: RCT. *BMJ* 2012; **344**: e3732.
13 Campbell KJ, Lioret S, McNaughton SA, Crawford DA, Salmon J, Ball K, *et al*. A parent-focused intervention to reduce infant obesity risk behaviors: a randomized trial. *Pediatrics* 2013; **13**: 652–660.
14 Certain LK, Kahn RS. Prevalence, correlates, and trajectory of TV viewing among infants and toddlers. *Pediatrics* 2002; **109**: 634–642.
15 Jackson DM, Djafarian K, Stewart J, Speakman JR. Increased TV viewing is associated with elevated body fatness but not with lower total energy expenditure in children. *Am J Clin Nutr* 2009; **89**: 1031–1036.
16 Bellissimo N, Pencharz PB, Thomas SG, Anderson GH. Effect of TV viewing at mealtime on food intake after a glucose preload in boys. *Pediatr Res* 2007; **61**: 745–749.
17 Taveras EM, McDonald J, O'Brien A, Haines J, Sherry B, Bottino CJ, *et al*. Healthy Habits, Happy Homes: Methods and baseline data of a randomized controlled trial to improve household routines for obesity prevention. *Prev Med* 2012; **55**: 418–426.
18 De Silva-Sanigorski AM, Bell AC, Kremer P, Nichols M, Crellin M, Smith M, *et al*. Reducing obesity in early childhood: results from Romp & Chomp, an Australian community wide intervention program. *Am J Clin Nutr* 2010; **91**: 831–840.
19 Canadian Society for Exercise Physiology. *Canadian physical activity and sedentary behaviour guidelines*, 2012. http://www.csep.ca/CMFiles/Guidelines/CSEP_Guidelines_Handbook.pdf (accessed October 2013).
20 Iglowstein I, Jenni OG, Molinari L, Largo RH. Sleep duration from infancy to adolescence: reference values and generational trends. *Pediatrics* 2003; **111**: 302–307.
21 Jimenez-Pavon D, Kelly J, Reilly JJ. Associations between objectively measured habitual physical activity and adiposity in children and adolescents: systematic review. *Int J Pediatr Obes* 2010; **5**: 3–18.

CHAPTER 5

Early physical activity and sedentary behaviours

Anthony D. Okely[1] and Xanne Janssen[2]

[1] Early Start Research Institute, University of Wollongong, Wollongong, Australia
[2] Physical Activity for Health Group, School of Psychological Sciences & Health, University of Strathclyde, Glasgow, UK

Introduction

Health professionals play a key role in promoting physical activity and limiting sitting and screen-time behaviour in the early years. When working with parents of young children, it is important for health professionals to understand the relationship of these behaviours to health outcomes, what evidence exists around the tracking of these behaviours from early childhood into childhood and adulthood, and on what evidence current physical activity and screen-time guidelines are based. This chapter summarises the evidence in these areas, based on a recent literature search of longitudinal and intervention studies (up to and including September 2013), and provides advice on promoting health-enhancing levels of these behaviours.

Physical activity, sedentary behaviour and health in the early years

Several studies have examined the impact of physical activity during the early years on health outcomes such as adiposity, musculoskeletal health, motor skill development and psychosocial health later in life. Seventy-seven per cent of the longitudinal studies examining the association between physical activity during the early years and adiposity later in life reported a negative association [1–10], whereas 23% of the studies reported no effect of physical activity on adiposity [11–13]. Randomised controlled trials examining the effect of an exercise programme on measures of adiposity did not report a significant effect [14–18]. However, the total duration of these studies was consistently shorter than the longitudinal studies. This may indicate that the beneficial effect of physical activity on adiposity levels may take longer to become noticeable.

Of the nine studies examining the association between physical activity and bone health [17, 19–26], 89% reported a positive association [17, 19–25]. Four studies examined the effect of passive extension and flexion range-of-motion exercises of the upper and lower extremities in premature infants [19, 21, 23, 24]. All reported a significant effect on bone strength after 4–8 weeks. Among pre-school-aged children, an increase in weight-bearing activities such as jumping and running, and moderate to vigorous

---

Early Years Nutrition and Healthy Weight, First Edition. Edited by Laura Stewart and Joyce Thompson.
© 2015 John Wiley & Sons, Ltd. Published 2015 by John Wiley & Sons, Ltd.

intensity physical activities (MVPA), was associated with better bone health during childhood [17, 20, 22, 25]. One cohort study reported that children with higher levels of physical activity at age 5 years showed greater agility and balance at age 6 years [13].

Six randomised controlled trials examined the effect of a movement skill intervention on pre-school children's motor skills; all reported greater improvements in those who received the intervention [14, 16, 18, 27–29]. In addition, one study reported that girls who received the intervention at age 4 years showed significantly better object-control skills compared to the control group. However, in boys the advantage noticed at the end of the intervention had disappeared by age 8 [29]. This may indicate that boys will participate in sports that help develop these skills during early childhood, whereas girls might engage less in these activities and need greater encouragement to participate to improve their motor skills.

The evidence on the beneficial effects of physical activity on cardio-metabolic health appears to be consistent. Eighty-six per cent of the studies reviewed reported significant differences in cardio-metabolic health outcomes during childhood between pre-school-aged children engaging in low levels of physical activity and highly active children [12, 13, 28, 30–32]. Physical activity during early childhood was also found to be associated with greater improvements in social and psychosocial outcomes such as social competence and internalising and externalising behavioural problems at later ages [27, 33, 34].

From the reported evidence, it can be concluded that physical activity during the early years is beneficial for adiposity, musculoskeletal health, cardio-metabolic health, psychosocial health and improved motor skill performance. For musculoskeletal health, motor skill performance and psychosocial health, these benefits appear to be short term, whereas the benefits for adiposity levels are apparent later in life. The evidence around the frequency and intensity of physical activity required for these health benefits is limited [35, 36]. Several recent cross-sectional studies have examined the impact of different intensities of physical activity on pre-school-aged children's health. These have shown that MVPA was associated with lower levels of adiposity, although no association for light intensity physical activity was evident [37–41]. Still, it remains unclear how the intensity of physical activity is related to health outcomes other than adiposity such as cardio-metabolic and psychosocial health outcomes [35, 36]. In addition, evidence on the dose (e.g. frequency and duration) of physical activity required for optimal development and health in pre-school-aged children is virtually non-existent. Table 5.1 summarises the evidence on the associations between physical activity and health outcomes.

Sedentary behaviour is defined as any activity with an energy expenditure value of less than or equal to 1.5 times resting metabolic rate (RMR) while in a sitting or reclining position. As such, sedentary behaviour is distinct from physical inactivity [42]. Among pre-school-aged children, screen behaviours such as television viewing are typically the most common, but not the only sedentary behaviours [43]. Pre-school-aged children can also be sedentary during motorised transport, while reading books, eating meals or engaging in art and craft activities. Children's total sedentary behaviour is therefore comprised of many different behaviours and it may be the overall volume of sedentariness and the length of the bout which are related to health outcomes.

Over the last decade, there has been an increase in the number of studies examining the association between sedentary behaviour and health. However, most of the studies reviewed for this chapter focused on the associations between screen time and health outcomes. Eighty-seven per cent of the studies that examined the association between screen time during the early years and adiposity later in life found a positive association

Table 5.1 Association between physical activity and health outcomes.

Outcome	Associated with physical activity		Not associated with physical activity	Summary coding	
	References	Association (+/−)		n/N (%)	Association* (+/−)
Adiposity	1–10	−	11–18	10/18 (55.6)	?
Musculoskeletal health	17, 19–25	+		12/12 (100)	++
Motor development	13, 14, 16, 18, 27–29	+		7/7 (100)	++
Cardiovascular health	12, 13, 28, 30–32	+	5	6/7 (85.7)	++
Psychosocial health	27, 33, 34	+		3/3 (100)	+

*0, no association (support from 0 to 33% of studies); ?, indeterminate or inconsistent association (34–59%); +, positive association; −, negative association (60–100% of studies). When four or more studies support an association or no association, the association is coded as 00, ++, or −−.

[2, 8, 44–53]. Thirteen per cent did not report significant effects of sedentary behaviour on adiposity; however, children with higher levels of television (TV) viewing were more likely to be overweight or have an increase in body mass index (BMI) [54, 55]. In addition, one study suggested that it was not the sedentary aspect of television viewing that contributed to the increase in BMI but the exposure to energy-dense food and beverage advertisements on TV [56].

One study found that children who spent less than 2 hours watching TV had better measures of bone health [57]. One study examining the effect of sedentary behaviour on motor development reported that each additional 1.2 hours of parent-reported TV time at 29 months of age predicted lower motor locomotion scores at 65 months [58]. Two studies reported on the effect of TV viewing on cardio-metabolic outcomes. These found that young children who spent more time watching TV were less fit and had higher levels of cholesterol than children who spent less time watching TV [47, 50]. In addition, pre-school-aged children who watched more than 2 hours of TV a day were 1.8 times more likely to experience asthmatic symptoms at the age of 11.5 years [59]. All studies examining the association between TV viewing and psychosocial health outcomes such as hyperactivity, social behaviour, victimisation and bullying reported significant adverse effects [50, 60–64]. In addition, watching violent and/or non-educational programmes resulted in an increased risk of poor psychosocial health outcomes [63, 64]. Sixty-six per cent of the studies reported that early TV viewing was associated with attention problems later in life [65, 66].

Sixty per cent of the studies reviewed found that exposure to TV viewing during the infant and toddler period resulted in lower levels of language, reading skills and mathematics achievement at ages 1.5–10 years [50, 63–65, 67–69]. Twenty per cent reported no association between TV viewing and children's reading or language development [50, 70], whereas another 20% of the studies reported no effect of educational TV programmes on children's language development [69, 71]. One cohort study examining the association between sedentary and dietary behaviours found that for each additional hour of TV viewing at 29 months of age, children were 16% more likely to have lower levels of fruit and vegetable intake by 10 years of age, and 9 and 10% more likely to have higher consumption of soft drinks and snacks, respectively [50].

Table 5.2 Association between screen time and health outcomes.

Outcome	Associated with screen time		Not associated with screen time	Summary coding	
	References	Association (+/−)		n/N(%)	Association* (+/−)
Adiposity	2, 8, 44–53, 56	+	54, 55	13/15 (86.7%)	++
Musculoskeletal health	57	−		1/1 (100%)	−
Motor development	58	−		1/1 (100%)	−
Cardiovascular health	47, 50, 59	−		3/3 (100%)	−
Psychosocial health	50, 60–66	−	74	8/9 (88.9%)	−−
Cognitive development	50[†], 63–65, 67–69	−	69–71	7/10 (70%)	−−
Poor dietary behaviours	50	+		1/1 (100%)	+

*0, no association (support from 0 to 33% of studies); ?, indeterminate or inconsistent association (34–59%); +, positive association; −, negative association (60–100% of studies). When four or more studies support an association or no association, the association is coded as 00, ++, or −−.

†Screen time was associated with maths achievement but not with reading or language development.

As mentioned previously, TV viewing is only one component of sedentary behaviour. The association between health outcomes and TV viewing might be mediated by other factors, such as dietary behaviours, which have been found to be associated with TV viewing [72] as well as exposure to advertisements [56]. The evidence around total sedentary behaviour and health outcomes in young children is lacking [37, 73]. Nevertheless, it is clear that TV viewing is associated with unfavourable levels of adiposity, psychosocial health and cognitive development. As with physical activity, it appears that the effect of sedentary behaviour during the early years on adiposity surfaces later in life, while the negative effects of screen time on psychosocial health and cognitive development are noticeable immediately and continue into childhood. Table 5.2 summarises the evidence on the associations between sedentary behaviour and health outcomes.

Tracking of physical activity and sedentary behaviour

The degree to which physical activity and sedentary behaviour change over time is often referred to as 'tracking'. Only a small number of studies have examined how physical activity tracks from the early years into childhood and adulthood. These have been recently reviewed and show that physical activity and sedentary behaviour track at a moderate level (mean tracking coefficients of 0.39 and 0.49, respectively), which means they stay relatively stable from early childhood into childhood [75].

Recommendations on levels of physical activity

Since 2010, Australia, UK and Canada have released government-endorsed national guidelines for physical activity in the early years [76–78]. In 2009, the National Association of Sport and Physical Education (NASPE) in the USA released the second edition of *Active Start: A Statement of Physical Activity Guidelines for Children from Birth to Age 5* [79]. Other organisations such as the Institute of Medicine in the USA have published specific recommendations for obesity prevention in early childhood [80]. Embedded in

Table 5.3 Summary of existing physical activity guidelines/recommendations for the early years.

Country	Organisation	Date	Ages (years)	Summary of guideline/recommendations
USA	National Association for Sport and Physical Education (NASPE)	2009 (2nd edition)	0–5	Infants should interact with caregivers in daily physical activities that are dedicated to exploring movement and the environment Toddlers should engage in at least 30 minutes of structured physical activity and at least 60 minutes – and up to several hours daily – of unstructured physical activity per day Pre-school-aged children should accumulate at least 60 minutes structured physical activity and should engage in at least 60 minutes – and up to several hours – of unstructured physical activity each day
Australia	Australian Government Department of Health and Ageing	2010	0–5	For healthy development in infants, physical activity – particularly supervised floor-based play in safe environments – should be encouraged from birth Toddlers and pre-school-aged children should be physically active every day for at least 3 hours, spread throughout the day
UK	Department of Health	2011	0–5	Physical activity should be encouraged from birth, particularly through floor-based play and water-based activities in safe environments Children of pre-school age who are capable of walking unaided should be physically active daily for at least 180 minutes (3 hours), spread throughout the day
Canada	Canadian Society for Exercise Physiology (CSEP)	2012	0–4	Infants (aged <1 year) should be physically active several times daily particularly through interactive floor based play Toddlers (aged 1–2 years) and pre-school-aged children (aged 3–4 years) should accumulate at least 180 minutes of physical activity at any intensity spread throughout the day, including: • A variety of activities in different environments • Activities that develop movement skills • Progression toward at least 60 minutes of energetic play by 5 years of age
USA	Institute of Medicine (Child care specific)	2011	0–5	Infants should be provided with opportunities each day to move and explore their environments, including 'tummy time' for infants <6 months of age Toddlers and pre-school-aged children should be provided with opportunities for light, moderate and vigorous physical activity for at least 15 minutes/hour while children are in care

this publication were specific physical activity recommendations for child care services. A summary of these guidelines and recommendations is shown in Table 5.3.

There is a consistency in the guidelines from Australia, Canada and the UK. All three countries recommend toddlers and pre-school-aged children accumulate at least 3 hours of physical activity, spread throughout the day. It is important to note that, unlike the guidelines for school-aged children and young people, this activity does not need to be of a particular intensity (e.g. MVPA) to be beneficial. It is the amount of physical activity and the nature of it (predominantly physical activity play) that are important. This aligns with the natural activity patterns of young children which are characterised by short intense bursts of activity intermixed with periods of rest or lower intensity activity.

All five guidelines recommend that physical activity is an important part of healthy infant development and should be encouraged from birth. Parents and caregivers should be advised to interact in a physically active way as often as possible with their infant and provide a safe environment for them to explore. 'Tummy time' and floor-based play are specifically mentioned as the preferred types of physical activity for infants who are not yet walking.

Recommendations on levels of screen-based entertainment

Australia and Canada [81] have published guidelines relating to screen-based entertainment for the early years. In October 2013, the American Academy of Pediatrics updated their policy statement on 'Children, Adolescents, and the Media' [82]. The Institute of Medicine has also published recommendations for screen time for toddlers and pre-school-aged children as part of their 'Early Childhood Obesity Prevention Policies' document [80]. This includes specific recommendations for screen time during child care. A summary of these recommendations appears in Table 5.4.

Australia, Canada and the American Academy of Pediatrics all recommend that children under the age of 2 years should not spend any time watching TV or engaging with other screen-based entertainment. They also recommend less than 1 hour/day for children aged older than 2 years.

In addition to the recommendations were several important 'companion statements'. These were designed to provide supporting advice in specific areas such as not placing screen-based devices in children's bedrooms and enforcing family rules around not using screen-based devices at mealtimes and before bedtimes.

Recommendations on levels of sedentary behaviour

In recent years, sedentary behaviour recommendations have been broadened beyond screen-based entertainment to include other types of sedentary behaviour, specifically any that involve sitting or lying for extended periods. This is based on evidence in adults that total sitting and sitting for prolonged periods have a deleterious effect on some cardio-metabolic health outcomes [83].

Although there is not yet evidence linking total time and prolonged sitting with adverse health outcomes in young children, many countries and jurisdictions have made recommendations in this area. The rationale for this is twofold. Firstly, it is not developmentally appropriate for young children to sit or be restrained for long periods of time. Secondly, many of the cardio-metabolic risk factors linked with total and prolonged sitting in adults have their genesis in early childhood and these risk factors also 'track' from childhood into adulthood [84]. A summary of the recommendations relating to sitting time in the early years is shown in Table 5.5.

All recommendations support the notion that it is not developmentally appropriate for young children to be sedentary for long periods of time. The maximum length of time is 1 hour and this includes not restraining young children in a car seat, stroller or high chair. It does not include sleeping, which is not classed as a sedentary behaviour according to the internationally accepted definition [42].

It is important to note that the term 'sedentary' is used in the NASPE (US), Australian, Canadian and UK guidelines. This terminology is consistent with guidelines for

Table 5.4 Summary of existing screen-based entertainment guidelines for the early years.

Country	Organisation	Date	Age (years)	Guideline/recommendations
USA	American Academy of Pediatrics	2013 (2nd edition)	NS*	Limit the amount of total entertainment screen time to <1–2 hours/day Discourage screen media exposure for children <2 years of age
Australia	Australian Government Department of Health and Ageing	2010	0–5	Children younger than 2 years of age should not spend any time watching television or using other electronic media (DVDs, computer and other electronic games) For children 2–5 years of age, sitting and watching television and the use of other electronic media (DVDs, computer and other electronic games) should be limited to <1 hour/day
Canada	Canadian Society for Exercise Physiology (CSEP)	2012	0–4	For those under 2 years of age, screen time (e.g. television, computer, electronic games) is not recommended For children 2–4 years of age, screen time should be limited to under, 1 hour/day; less is better
USA	Institute of Medicine	2011	2–5	Child care settings should limit screen time, including television, cell phone or digital media, for pre-school-aged children (aged 2–5 years) to <30 minutes/day for children in half-day programmes or <1 hour/day for those in full-day programmes Adults working with children should limit screen time, including television, cell phone or digital media, to <2 hours/day for children aged 2–5 years

*NS, not specified. However, guidelines target children and adolescents and there is a specific guideline for children younger than 2 years.

Table 5.5 Summary of existing sedentary behaviour guidelines related to sitting time in the early years.

Country	Organisation	Date	Age (years)	Guideline/recommendations
USA	National Association for Sport and Physical Education (NASPE)	2009 (2nd edition)	0–5	Toddlers and pre-school-aged children should not be sedentary for >60 minutes at a time except when sleeping
Australia	Australian Government Department of Health and Ageing	2010	0–5	Infants, toddlers and pre-school-aged children should not be sedentary, restrained, or kept inactive, for >1 hour at a time, with the exception of sleeping
UK	Department of Health	2010	0–5	All children under 5 years should minimise the amount of time spent being sedentary (being restrained or sitting) for extended periods (except time spent sleeping)
Canada	Canadian Society for Exercise Physiology (CSEP)	2012	0–4	For healthy growth and development, caregivers should minimise the time infants, toddlers and pre-school-aged children spend being sedentary during waking hours. This includes prolonged sitting or being restrained (e.g. stroller, high chair) for >1 hour at a time
USA	Institute of Medicine	2011	2–5	Child care services should implement activities for toddlers and pre-school-aged children that limit sitting or standing to no >30 minutes at a time

children, young people and adults, and better encapsulates the intensity in which these two behaviours are undertaken. It also minimises confusion with other terms such as 'sitting' which is a posture in which sedentary behaviours are commonly undertaken but also one which some physical activities such as riding a bicycle can be performed.

The Institute of Medicine (USA) recommendation differs somewhat from the others. Whilst it does recommend limiting the amount of time young people spend sitting during child care hours, and not restraining their movement (which is consistent with the other guidelines), it includes 'standing' in both the recommendation and suggested potential actions. The inclusion of standing is not consistent with the other guidelines and is not consistent with the definition of sedentary behaviour which only includes sitting and lying postures [42]. This is based on evidence in adults that sitting and standing have different effects on cardio-metabolic health [85].

Summary of recommendations

A review of the current guidelines for physical activity, screen-based entertainment and sedentary behaviour shows that there are several countries and organisations that have developed guidelines for the early years. This is a positive sign and recognises the unique developmental characteristics and needs of children over the first 4–5 years of life. It is recommended that other countries and international jurisdictions (such as the European Union and World Health Organization) also develop specific guidelines for the early years to add to their existing guidelines for school-aged-children and adults.

Parents and carers, early childhood settings, primary care physicians or general practitioners, and paediatricians are important in encouraging and promoting these recommendations. All the cues for physical activity and sedentary behaviour for children of this age are provided by their parents and carers. Parents should allow plenty of opportunities for unstructured play and aim for a balance between activities that encourage independence and appropriate risk taking (e.g. walking along a low wall), while maintaining a safe and supervised environment. As parents are important role models, they can help foster their child's involvement in and enjoyment of physical activity and play, and can also benefit their own health. They should look to interact in a gentle, physically active way with their infant, toddler or pre-school aged-child as often as possible.

As trusted sources of health information and advice, general practitioners and paediatricians can advocate for promotion of physical activity and limiting of screen-based sedentary behaviour in the home, early childhood setting and local communities. Along with other child health professionals, they can routinely ask parents how much time their young child spends being physically active (or even playing outdoors) and watching TV or using electronic media and advice on the health benefits and consequences of these behaviours, for both the child and the parent.

Conclusion

Physical activity during the first 5 years of life has important short- and long-term health benefits. Moreover, it has a role in facilitating the development of movement patterns and competence. Movement is the substrate of physical activity that is a basic human dimension and essential for children during the early years of life. Movement development, through exploration, learning and interacting with environments and other individuals must be encouraged and provided. There are many opportunities for young children to spend excessive times in sedentary behaviour, especially in screen-based entertainment, which can have deleterious effects on their health and development. These must be limited and replaced with more active options. The guidelines summarised in this chapter are based on the best available evidence and provide consistent advice on the amount of physical activity, screen-based entertainment and sedentary behaviour recommended for the early years.

Putting the evidence into practice

Promoting physical activity in a child care setting

Child care services have a key role in contributing to toddlers and pre-school-aged children meeting the physical activity and sedentary behaviour recommendations. Child care settings should encourage toddlers and pre-school-aged children to explore and play in both their indoor and outdoor environments. Although it is preferable that children be given access to space and equipment in an outdoor environment, many activities can also be undertaken in restricted outdoor environments (such as verandas and yards) and in indoor environments. Parents should select child care providers who promote physical activity and have adequate space, equipment and staff-to-child ratios in accordance with their regulatory requirements and quality assurance systems. Some specific, evidence-based actions that could be undertaken in child care to promote physical activity and reduce sedentary behaviour include the following:

- Providing a time each day for children to participate in some form of structured physical activity that is focused on developing their fundamental or gross motor skills. Improving gross motor skills has been shown to be effective in increasing the amount of time spent in physical activity up to 26 minutes/day during child care hours [18].
- Breaking up children's sedentary time through activity breaks incorporated at regular intervals throughout the day. A pilot study testing the strategy of incorporating five, 3-minute active 'energy breaks' throughout the day showed that, over a 3 week period, time spent in MVPA increased by 10 minutes/day and time spent sitting decreased by 12 minutes/day.
- Integrating physical activity with other learning areas. Evidence suggests that learning tasks involving gross motor movement can improve behavioural self-regulatory skills, which are required for concentration and attention and predict better school readiness [86, 87]. A pilot study conducted by Trost and colleagues [88] randomly assigned two classrooms to a programme integrating gross motor movement into mathematics, language, social studies and science activities, with educators integrating two activities of at least 10 minutes every half-day over 8 weeks. Compared with control (usual curriculum) children, intervention children spent significantly more time in MVPA per day (around 4 minutes) and showed higher levels of physical and verbal self-regulation.

How a health professional can advise parents about reducing screen time

Tom, a 4-year-old overweight boy, visits a dietitian with his parents. As a health professional, she explains to the parents why it is important that Tom limits the time he is sitting still or engaging in screen-based behaviours. Two main questions recommended by the American Academy of Pediatrics [82] that should be asked are (1) How much recreational screen time does your pre-school-aged child consume daily? (2) Is there a

TV set or an internet-connected electronic device in the child's bedroom? If the parents report that Tom spends more than 1 hour a day on screen-based behaviours, provide examples on how to reduce this. This would include turning the TV off during meal times, taking the TV out of the bedroom, providing alternative activities for Tom to do and setting rules around how and when screen time is allowed. During the next visit, follow-up with the parents on whether or not they were successful in reducing screen time.

TAKE HOME MESSAGES

- Physical activity during the early years is beneficial for health outcomes later in life.
- At least 180 minutes of physical activity per day is recommended; however, more is better.
- Higher intensity physical activities such as running and jumping have more beneficial effects compared with lower intensity physical activity (walking), especially for bone health and adiposity.
- Limit the time toddlers and pre-school-aged children spend using screen-based entertainment to less than 1 hour/day and limit the time young children are kept restrained.

References

1 Atkin AJ, Ekelund U, Møller NC, *et al.* Sedentary time in children: influence of accelerometer processing on health relations. *Med Sci Sports Exerc.* 2012; **45**: 1097–1104.
2 Jago R, Baranowski T, Baranowski JC, *et al.* BMI from 3–6 y of age is predicted by TV viewing and physical activity, not diet. *Int J Obes.* 2005; **29**: 557–564.
3 Klesges RC, Klesges LM, Eck LH, *et al.* A longitudinal analysis of accelerated weight gain in preschool children. *Pediatrics.* 1995; **95**: 126–130.
4 Ku L, Shapiro L, Crawford P, *et al.* Body composition and physical activity in 8-year-old children. *Am J Clin Nutr.* 1981; **34**: 2770–2775.
5 Metcalf BS, Jeffery AN, Hosking J, *et al.* Objectively measured physical activity and its association with adiponectin and other novel metabolic markers a longitudinal study in children (EarlyBird 38). *Diabetes Care.* 2009; **32**: 468–473.
6 Moore LL, Gao D, Bradlee ML, *et al.* Does early physical activity predict body fat change throughout childhood? *Prev Med.* 2003; **37**: 10–17.
7 Moore LL, Nguyen US, Rothman KJ, *et al.* Preschool physical activity level and change in body fatness in young children: the Framingham Children's Study. *Am J Epidemiol.* 1995; **142**: 982–988.
8 Sugimori H, Yoshida K, Izuno T, *et al.* Analysis of factors that influence body mass index from ages 3 to 6 years: a study based on the Toyama cohort study. *Pediatr Int.* 2004; **46**: 302–310.
9 Wells JC, Ritz P. Physical activity at 9–12 months and fatness at 2 years of age. *Am J Hum Biol.* 2001; **13**: 384–389.
10 Remmers T, Sleddens E, Gubbels J, *et al.* Relationship between physical activity and the development of BMI in children. *Med Sci Sports Exerc.* 2014; **46**: 177–184.
11 Li R, O'Connor L, Buckley D, *et al.* Relation of activity levels to body fat in infants 6 to 12 months of age. *J Pediatr.* 1995; **126**: 353–357.
12 Metcalf BS, Voss LD, Hosking J, *et al.* Physical activity at the government-recommended level and obesity-related health outcomes: a longitudinal study (Early Bird 37). *Arch Dis Child.* 2008; **93**: 772–777.
13 Bürgi F, Meyer U, Granacher U, *et al.* Relationship of physical activity with motor skills, aerobic fitness and body fat in preschool children: a cross-sectional and longitudinal study (Ballabeina). *Int J Obes.* 2011; **35**: 937–944.
14 Krombholz H. The impact of a 20-month physical activity intervention in child care centers on motor performance and weight in overweight and healthy-weight preschool children. *Percept Mot Skills.* 2012; **115**: 919–932.
15 Mo-suwan L, Pongprapai S, Junjana C, *et al.* Effects of a controlled trial of a school-based exercise program on the obesity indexes of preschool children. *Am J Clin Nutr.* 1998; **68**: 1006–1011.
16 Reilly JJ, Kelly L, Montgomery C, *et al.* Physical activity to prevent obesity in young children: cluster randomised controlled trial. *BMJ.* 2006; **333**: 1041.

17   Specker B, Binkley T. Randomized trial of physical activity and calcium supplementation on bone mineral content in 3-to-5 year-old children. *J Bone Miner Res.* 2003; **18**; 885–892.

18   Jones RA, Riethmuller A, Hesketh K, *et al.* Promoting fundamental movement skill development and physical activity in early childhood settings: a cluster randomized controlled trial. *Pediatr Exerc Sci.* 2011; **23**: 600–615.

19   Aly H, Moustafa MF, Hassanein SM, *et al.* Physical activity combined with massage improves bone mineralization in premature infants: a randomized trial. *J Perinatol.* 2004; **24**: 305–309.

20   Casazza K, Hanks L, Hidalgo B, *et al.* Short-term physical activity intervention decreases femoral bone marrow adipose tissue in young children: a pilot study. *Bone.* 2012; **50**: 23–27.

21   Chen HL, Lee CL, Tseng HI, *et al.* Assisted exercise improves bone strength in very low birthweight infants by bone quantitative ultrasound. *J Paediatr Child Health.* 2010; **46**: 653–659.

22   Janz KF, Letuchy EM, Gilmore JME, *et al.* Early physical activity provides sustained bone health benefits later in childhood. *Med Sci Sports Exerc.* 2010; **42**: 1072–1078.

23   Litmanovitz I, Dolfin T, Arnon S, *et al.* Assisted exercise and bone strength in preterm infants. *Calcif Tissue Int.* 2007; **80**: 39–43.

24   Litmanovitz I, Dolfin T, Friedland O, *et al.* Early physical activity intervention prevents decrease of bone strength in very low birth weight infants. *Pediatrics.* 2003; **112**: 15–19.

25   Specker B. Nutrition influences bone development from infancy through toddler years. *J Nutr.* 2004; **134**: 691S–695S.

26   Specker BL, Mulligan L, Ho M. Longitudinal study of calcium intake, physical activity, and bone mineral content in infants 6–18 months of age. *J Bone Miner Res.* 1999; **14**: 569–576.

27   Porter LS. The impact of physical-physiological activity on infants' growth and development. *Nurs Res.* 1972; **21**: 210–219.

28   Puder J, Marques-Vidal P, Schindler C, *et al.* Effect of multidimensional lifestyle intervention on fitness and adiposity in predominantly migrant preschool children (Ballabeina): cluster randomised controlled trial. *BMJ.* 2011; **343**: d6195.

29   Zask A, Adams JK, Brooks LO, *et al.* Tooty Fruity Vegie: an obesity prevention intervention evaluation in Australian preschools. *Health Promot J Austr.* 2012; **23**: 10–15.

30   Alpert B, Field TM, Goldstein S, *et al.* Aerobics enhances cardiovascular fitness and agility in preschoolers. *Health Psychol.* 1990; **9**: 48–56.

31   Sääkslahti A, Numminen P, Varstala V, *et al.* Physical activity as a preventive measure for coronary heart disease risk factors in early childhood. *Scand J Med Sci Sports.* 2004; **14**: 143–149.

32   Shea S, Basch CE, Gutin B, *et al.* The rate of increase in blood pressure in children 5 years of age is related to changes in aerobic fitness and body mass index. *Pediatrics.* 1994; **94**: 465–470.

33   Buss DM, Block JH, Block J. Preschool activity level: personality correlates and developmental implications. *Child Dev.* 1980; **51**: 401–408.

34   Lobo YB, Winsler A. The effects of a creative dance and movement program on the social competence of head start preschoolers. *Soc Dev.* 2006; **15**: 501–519.

35   Timmons BW, Naylor P-J, Pfeiffer KA. Physical activity for preschool children—how much and how? *Can J Public Health.* 2007; **98**: S122–S134.

36   Timmons BW, Leblanc AG, Carson V, *et al.* Systematic review of physical activity and health in the early years (aged 0–4 years). *Appl Physiol Nutr Metab.* 2012; **37**: 773–792.

37   Collings PJ, Brage S, Ridgway CL, *et al.* Physical activity intensity, sedentary time, and body composition in preschoolers. *Am J Clin Nutr.* 2013; **97**: 1020–1028.

38   Metallinos-Katsaras ES, Freedson PS, Fulton JE, *et al.* The association between an objective measure of physical activity and weight status in preschoolers. *Obesity.* 2007; **15**: 686–694.

39   Janz KF, Levy SM, Burns TL, *et al.* Fatness, physical activity, and television viewing in children during the adiposity rebound period: the Iowa Bone Development Study. *Prev Med.* 2002; **35**: 563–571.

40   Vale SMCG, Santos RMR, Soares-Miranda LMdC, *et al.* Objectively measured physical activity and body mass index in preschool children. *Int J Pediatr.* 2010; **2010**: 1–6.

41   Davies D. *Child Development, Third Edition: A Practitioner's Guide.* Guilford Publications: New York, 2010.

42   Sedentary Behaviour Research Network. Standardised use of the terms 'sedentary' and 'sedentary behaviours': letter to the editor. *Appl Physiol Nutr Metab.* 2012; **37**: 540–542.

43   LeBlanc AG, Spence JC, Carson V, *et al.* Systematic review of sedentary behaviour and health indicators in the early years (aged 0–4 years). *Appl Physiol Nutr Metab.* 2012; **37**: 753–772.

44   Blair NJ, Thompson JM, Black PN, *et al.* Risk factors for obesity in 7-year-old European children: the Auckland Birthweight Collaborative Study. *Arch Dis Child.* 2007; **92**: 866–871.

45 Brown JE, Broom DH, Nicholson JM, *et al.* Do working mothers raise couch potato kids? Maternal employment and children's lifestyle behaviours and weight in early childhood. *Soc Sci Med.* 2010; **70**: 1816–1824.

46 Francis LA, Lee Y, Birch LL. Parental weight status and girls' television viewing, snacking, and body mass indexes. *Obes Res.* 2003; **11**: 143–151.

47 Hancox RJ, Milne BJ, Poulton R. Association between child and adolescent television viewing and adult health: a longitudinal birth cohort study. *The Lancet.* 2004; **364**: 257–262.

48 Intusoma U, Mo-suwan L, Ruangdaraganon N, *et al.* Effect of television viewing on social–emotional competence of young Thai children. *Infant Behav Dev.* 2013; **36**: 679–685.

49 Lumeng JC, Rahnama S, Appugliese D, *et al.* Television exposure and overweight risk in preschoolers. *Arch Pediatr Adolesc Med.* 2006; **160**: 417–422.

50 Pagani LS, Fitzpatrick C, Barnett TA, *et al.* Prospective associations between early childhood television exposure and academic, psychosocial, and physical well-being by middle childhood. *Arch Pediatr Adolesc Med.* 2010; **164**: 425–431.

51 Proctor M, Moore L, Gao D, *et al.* Television viewing and change in body fat from preschool to early adolescence: the Framingham Children's Study. *Int J Obes.* 2003; **27**: 827–833.

52 Reilly JJ, Armstrong J, Dorosty AR, *et al.* Early life risk factors for obesity in childhood: cohort study. *BMJ.* 2005; **330**: 1357.

53 Wijga AH, Scholtens S, Bemelmans WJ, *et al.* Diet, screen time, physical activity, and childhood overweight in the general population and in high risk subgroups: prospective analyses in the PIAMA birth cohort. *J Obes.* 2010; **2010**: 1–9.

54 Balaban G, Motta M, Silva G. Early weaning and other potential risk factors for overweight among preschool children. *Clinics.* 2010; **65**: 181–187.

55 Dennison BA, Russo TJ, Burdick PA, *et al.* An intervention to reduce television viewing by preschool children. *Arch Pediatr Adolesc Med.* 2004; **158**: 170–176.

56 Zimmerman FJ, Bell JF. Associations of television content type and obesity in children. *Am J Public Health.* 2010; **100**: 334–340.

57 Wosje KS, Khoury PR, Claytor RP, *et al.* Adiposity and TV viewing are related to less bone accrual in young children. *J Pediatr.* 2009; **154**: 79–85.

58 Pagani LS, Fitzpatrick C, Barnett TA. Early childhood television viewing and kindergarten entry readiness. *Pediatr Res.* 2013; **74**: 350–355.

59 Sherriff A, Maitra A, Ness AR, *et al.* Association of duration of television viewing in early childhood with the subsequent development of asthma. *Thorax.* 2009; **64**: 321–325.

60 Zimmerman FJ, Glew GM, Christakis DA, *et al.* Early cognitive stimulation, emotional support, and television watching as predictors of subsequent bullying among grade-school children. *Arch Pediatr Adolesc Med.* 2005; **159**: 384–388.

61 Mistry KB, Minkovitz CS, Strobino DM, *et al.* Children's television exposure and behavioral and social outcomes at 5.5 years: does timing of exposure matter? *Pediatrics.* 2007; **120**: 762–769.

62 Cheng S, Maeda T, Yoichi S, *et al.* Early television exposure and children's behavioral and social outcomes at age 30 months. *J Epidemiol.* 2010; **20**: S482–S489.

63 Tomopoulos S, Dreyer BP, Valdez P, *et al.* Media content and externalizing behaviors in Latino toddlers. *Ambul Pediatr.* 2007; **7**: 232–238.

64 Christakis DA, Zimmerman FJ. Violent television viewing during preschool is associated with anti-social behavior during school age. *Pediatrics.* 2007; **120**: 993–999.

65 Zimmerman FJ, Christakis DA. Children's television viewing and cognitive outcomes: a longitudinal analysis of national data. *Arch Pediatr Adolesc Med.* 2005; **159**: 619–625.

66 Christakis DA, Zimmerman FJ, DiGiuseppe DL, *et al.* Early television exposure and subsequent attentional problems in children. *Pediatrics.* 2004; **113**: 708–713.

67 Chonchaiya W, Pruksananonda C. Television viewing associates with delayed language development. *Acta Paediatr.* 2008; **97**: 977–982.

68 Alston E, James-Roberts IS. Home environments of 10-month-old infants selected by the WILSTAAR screen for pre-language difficulties. *Int J Lang Commun Disord.* 2005; **40**: 123–136.

69 Richert RA, Robb MB, Fender JG, *et al.* Word learning from baby videos. *Arch Pediatr Adolesc Med.* 2010; **164**: 432–437.

70 Schmidt ME, Rich M, Rifas-Shiman SL, *et al.* Television viewing in infancy and child cognition at 3 years of age in a US cohort. *Pediatrics.* 2009; **123**: e370–e375.

71 Robb MB, Richert RA, Wartella EA. Just a talking book? Word learning from watching baby videos. *Brit J Dev Psychol.* 2009; **27**: 27–45.

72 Pearson N, Biddle SJH. Sedentary behavior and dietary intake in children, adolescents, and adults: a systematic review. *Am J Prev Med.* 2011; **41**: 178–188.

73 Byun W, Liu J, Pate R. Association between objectively measured sedentary behavior and body mass index in preschool children. *Int J Obes.* 2013; **37**: 961–965.

74 Foster EM, Watkins S. The value of reanalysis: TV viewing and attention problems. *Child Dev.* 2010; **81**: 368–375.

75 Jones RA, Hinkley T, Okely AD, *et al.* Tracking physical activity and sedentary behaviour in childhood: a systematic review. *Am J Prev Med.* 2013; **44**: 651–658.

76 Australian Government, Department of Health and Ageing. *Move and Play Every Day. National Physical Activity Recommendations for Children 0–5 Years.* http://www.health.gov.au/internet/main/publishing. nsf/Content/npra-0-5yrs-brochure (accessed 23 July 2013).

77 Chief Medical Officers. *Start Active, Stay Active: A Report on Physical Activity for Health from the Four Home Countries'.* http://www.gov.uk/government/publications/start-active-stay-active-a-report-on-physical-activity-from-the-four-home-countries-chief-medical-officers (accessed 23 November 2013).

78 Canadian Society for Exercise Physiology. *Canadian Physical Activity Guidelines (Aged 0–4 Years).* http:// www.csep.ca/english/view.asp?x=949 (accessed 23 November 2013).

79 National Association for Sport and Physical Education (NASPE). *Active Start: A Statement of Physical Activity Guidelines for Children From Birth to Five Years.* NASPE: Reston, VA, 2000, 1–26.

80 Institute of Medicine of the National Academies. *Early Childhood Obesity Prevention Policies: Policies Goals, Recommendations, and Potential Actions.* National Academies Press: Washington, DC, 2011.

81 Canadian Society for Exercise Physiology. *Canadian Sedentary Behavior Guidelines (Aged 0–4 Years).* http://www.csep.ca/english/view.asp?x=949 (accessed 23 November 2013).

82 American Academy of Pediatrics. Children, Adolescents, and the Media. *Pediatrics.* 2013; **132**: 958–961.

83 Van Uffelen JG, Wong J, Chau JY, *et al.* Occupational sitting and health risks: a systematic review. *Am J Prev Med.* 2010; **39**: 379–388.

84 Berenson GS. Childhood risk factors predict adult risk associated with subclinical cardiovascular disease: the Bogalusa Heart Study. *Am J Cardiol.* 2002; **90**: L3–L7.

85 Hamilton MT, Hamilton DG, Zderic TW. Role of low energy expenditure and sitting in obesity, metabolic syndrome, type 2 diabetes, and cardiovascular disease. *Diabetes.* 2007; **56**: 2655–2667.

86 Diamond A, Lee K. Interventions shown to aid executive function development in children 4 to 12 years old. *Science.* 2011; **333**: 959–964.

87 Becker D, McClelland M, Loprinzi PD, *et al.* Physical activity, self-regulation, and early academic achievement in preschool children. *Early Educ Dev.* 2014; **25**: 56–70.

88 Trost SG, Fees B, Dzewaltowski D. Feasibility and efficacy of a 'move and learn' physical activity curriculum in preschool children. *J Phys Activ Health.* 2008; **5**: 88–103.

CHAPTER 6

Talking about weight with families

Paul Chadwick[1] and Helen Croker[2]

[1] Research Department of Clinical, Educational and Health Psychology, University College London, London, UK
[2] Department of Epidemiology and Public Health, University College London, London, UK

Introduction

Whilst 'overweight' and 'obesity' are medical terms, public understandings of these words, especially as they relate to children's growth and development, are complex. For many parents, a diagnosis of obesity carries with it a significant degree of stigma, shame and guilt. Such feelings can have a profound impact on how families respond to messages about the relationship between a child's weight and their health and how receptive they are to offers of intervention.

This chapter will describe the factors affecting families' understanding of overweight and obesity in children and explore what this means for health professionals looking to communicate effectively about this sensitive issue.

What makes childhood obesity a sensitive issue?

Whilst the size and rate of growth of a child is used as a marker of healthy or unhealthy development in most cultures, there is a great deal of variability in what meanings are given to particular body sizes and shapes. Historically, children who are perceived to be big for their age have been viewed as healthy and terms such as 'bonny' and 'chubby' are commonly used with affection and connote approval of healthy development for bigger babies and children. In countries with significant levels of deprivation and where food may be scarce, heavier children may be perceived as healthier since thinness is associated with disease and poverty. Meanings ascribed to the larger body extend beyond health and serve as cultural markers of socio-economic status. In some cultures, having a child that is larger than their peers is valued because it communicates the wealth and prosperity of a family (see Gilman [1] for a review of cultural meanings associated with body size).

Practitioners working amongst multicultural communities need to be sensitive to the range of meanings that can be attached to the overweight body. Nevertheless, attitudes towards the obese amongst majority populations in Westernised countries are generally negative, with heavier bodies being seen as aesthetically unappealing and indicating poor character or emotional dysfunction. This constellation of negative beliefs about and behaviours towards overweight and obese individuals has been

Early Years Nutrition and Healthy Weight, First Edition. Edited by Laura Stewart and Joyce Thompson.
© 2015 John Wiley & Sons, Ltd. Published 2015 by John Wiley & Sons, Ltd.

termed 'weight stigma' [2, 3] and provides the basis for sensitivities about a child's weight status. Weight stigma has been shown to negatively affect the life chances of overweight and obese adults such that they are less likely to achieve success academically, vocationally and domestically. Negative attitudes towards heavier individuals are frequently expressed as verbal abuse and may partly account for the development of poor body image typically experienced by overweight individuals [4]. Overweight and obese children experience high levels of weight-related teasing and bullying from an early age and this includes negative verbal commentary inside the home from family members, as well as in schools, clubs and friendship groups [5, 6]. Within the healthcare setting, overweight and obese adults report experiences of derogatory and discriminatory behaviour targeted at their size [3]. Similarly, parents of obese children report that health professionals can be rude, judgemental and dismissive about their concerns, often blaming parents as the primary cause of the excessive weight gain [7–10]. Such views are reinforced by inflammatory media coverage in which childhood obesity is often portrayed as consequence of poor or neglectful parenting.

The negative meanings ascribed to the technical terms 'overweight' and 'obesity' means that the process of identification and diagnosis is experienced by many parents as labelling children with an unwanted and stigmatised identity. Understandably, parents are resistant to such labelling out of a desire to protect children from the negative impact of weight stigma, which is perceived to damage a child's psychological well-being [11]. Overweight children often become overweight adults and may eventually become parents themselves. Such parents have experienced first-hand the impact of weight stigmatisation and its consequences. They may be especially sensitised to its presence and keenly motivated to protect their own children from its effects.

Given the importance of this concern it is surprising that there is little research on the actual impact of talking to children about their weight status. What few studies exist suggest that there is minimal harm associated with talking about a child's weight status if done in a sensitive manner [9, 12, 13]. Nevertheless, failure to find evidence of psychological harm does not mean that talking about weight may not be an emotionally challenging, difficult or occasionally distressing activity for parents, children and professionals. The degree to which parental experience and sensitivities will lead to a strong negative reaction to learning about the health implications of a child's size will vary. Nevertheless, it is important for practitioners working in this area to anticipate such sensitivity and to prepare to work constructively with it, rather than avoiding it, or wishing it away.

Perceptions of child obesity and the challenge of identification

The threshold at which a child's size crosses the boundary of a 'normal' variation in development into something that is harmful to health is largely invisible to most common-sense ways of understanding body size. Whilst most people base their judgements of the healthiness of a child's size by how they look, research has consistently shown that visual assessment, apart from at the more extreme ranges, is a poor indicator of a child's actual weight status. It has been estimated that as many as 65% of parents fail to correctly identify their children as being overweight or obese. The degree of misperception tends to be higher in parents of younger children (2–6 years) but becomes more accurate with increasing age [14]. The most likely explanation for this observation is that parents' visual reference points for what constitutes an unhealthy size have been distorted by the dramatic increase in the prevalence in obesity [15] and exposure to the extreme images commonly used to illustrate media reports about the condition [16]. Furthermore, parents make use of a variety of information when making judgements about whether their child's size has crossed the line into unhealthiness. They use markers such as clothing size and waist circumference when considering whether to take action or seek help and are more concerned with the health impact of the behaviours associated with obesity (poor diet and inactivity) than they are about a child's weight [16, 17]. Even if parents are aware that their child is overweight they tend not to act because of the commonly held belief that children grow out of any excess weight accumulated when young. It is also the case that the media often misreports and misrepresents population-based screening programmes to identify overweight children in ways that lead parents to question the value of diagnoses based on interpretations of body mass index (BMI).

Parents are active decision makers rather than passively ignorant about their child's development. However, the common sense reference points that parents use to make judgements about the health of their children's size are at odds with the relatively technical and counter-intuitive processes involved with medical identification. This can create a tension between medically defined diagnostic categories and lay perceptions. So, whilst there may be increasing professional consensus about the negative health consequences of childhood obesity and how to measure it, this should be set against a public that is currently wary of the issue and sceptical of the validity of the medical viewpoint.

The impact of screening programmes

One potentially useful response to the widespread confusion about body size are the population-based screening programmes implemented by some countries to help parents identify children whose weight carries health risks. These typically involve measuring children's weight and height in school and providing feedback regarding weight status to parents (e.g. [18]). These programmes appear to be acceptable to parents [12, 19, 20], students [21], schools and school nurses [22, 23]. Whilst few studies have evaluated their impact quantitatively [24], such programmes appear to increase parental recognition of child overweight [25, 26], with parents who receive personalised feedback reporting intentions to change child eating and activity behaviour [12, 25, 27]. Less is known about whether these intentions translate into actual behaviour change but work is underway examining this [28]. Not all parents are convinced by feedback indicating that their child is overweight; however, many see weight as less important than their child being happy, eating healthily and being active [29]. Whilst concerns have been raised over the potential of such screening programmes to cause harm, with stigmatisation, promotion of dieting, body dissatisfaction, and lowered self-esteem raised as potential consequences (e.g. [30]), the few data available have not borne this out [9, 12].

General principles of handling sensitive conversations

Although screening programmes appear to be effective at raising awareness in parents, it is also the case that coverage is largely limited to one point in a child's life and, anecdotally, parents of heavier children are more likely to opt out of the process although this appears to improve once programmes are established [31]. For these reasons, many overweight and obese children will be identified as being so by their parents, or during healthcare consultations about other matters. There is near universal acceptance that talking about children's weight is a difficult thing to do. Professionals, parents and children find talking about weight an uncomfortable subject, and very few feel sufficiently knowledgeable and skilled to have such conversations [13, 32]. General principles of family-centred care [33], communicating bad news and handling sensitive discussions [34] can be drawn upon to help professionals and family members work together for the health of the child. The UK Royal College of Nursing (RCN) provides a useful framework for supporting the communication of news that may be received negatively and can be adapted to help practitioners think about how to communicate about weight-related issues generally and the weight screening and feedback conversation specifically. The framework proposes that there are four phases to consider when delivering information about sensitive areas: *preparation* of the self, recipient and environment, the actual *communication* strategies used, *planning* and *follow-up*. Table 6.1 describes the issues to consider in each phase and illustrates how they might be applied to the weight feedback situation.

Establishing lines of communication
It is good practice when talking about sensitive issues with families to consider who needs to know what, and to be mindful of parents' wishes about what and how information is shared with their child. Some parents may not wish to discuss their children's weight status with the child present whereas others might feel this would reinforce existing concerns and build upon conversations that have already occurred within the family. It can be helpful to find an opportunity to ask the parent directly about how they want to proceed with the discussions. How easy this is to achieve will depend largely on the organisation of the setting in which the conversation is to happen, and how easy it is to organise care around this. Parents are often the best guide to what is appropriate to talk about with their child but they can often share some of the same prejudices and unhelpful ideas about overweight and obesity as the general public. It can be helpful to talk directly to the child to help parents develop a helpful way of communicating about weight-related issues.

Purposive use of language
There can be a lot of anxiety about what words are most appropriate to use when talking about a child's weight status. Health professionals have been observed to use euphemisms (i.e. large, heavy, big) rather than medical terms (e.g. obesity) in order to avoid offending and alienating families [35]. Parents have a wide range of views about what words are acceptable and helpful when talking about their children's weight status. Some express a strong dislike of the terms 'overweight' and 'obese' since they are perceived as labelling and stigmatising the child, whereas others think that the use of euphemisms minimises the seriousness of the condition [9, 11]. It has been suggested the use of medical terminology such as 'obesity' and 'overweight'

Table 6.1 Phases involved in constructing weight feedback conversations that are responsive to parental sensitivities.

Phase	Issues to consider	Application to the weight feedback situation
Preparation	Decide who you are going to talk to and what they need to know	Who needs to understand the child's weight status? What is the implication of the child's age and stage of development? Does the child have the emotional maturity and cognitive ability to discuss their weight and its implications? What are the parents' preferences for discussing weight-related matters in front of their children? How will information be passed to those who have the most influence on the child's eating and activity behaviours?
	Make sure you have the relevant history so as to be able to talk meaningfully about the news you are to deliver	What is the wider family history in relation to weight status? How might this affect how family members receive the news about their child's weight status? Is it possible to link the child's weight status to existing health-related concerns within the family?
	Rehearse delivering the news mentally, and practice with peers to get feedback about your knowledge and skills	Diagnosis of obesity using BMI charts is a complex technical task. Can you deliver an explanation succinctly and accurately that respects the diverse range of cognitive and intellectual abilities you are likely to encounter?
	Prepare the environment to make sure it is conducive to talking about a sensitive subject	Think about the environment in which you may wish to receive news about a sensitive issue. Environments which are private and where communication can be face-to face are optimal. If face-to-face contact is not possible then how can you create an environment that allows respectful and private conversation?
Communication	Explore what is understood by the parent already	Ask parents what they understand about the reason for the screening procedure, and whether they have any views about the likely outcome.
	Give information honestly, but with sensitivity.	Avoid use of euphemisms when talking about medical categorisation but acknowledge the discomfort that medical terminology such as the words 'obese' and 'overweight' can cause. Do not overuse such terms once the meanings and implications are understood
	Use simple language and avoid medical jargon where possible	Use visual aids such as BMI charts to support explanations of how children's current and projected weight status may affect their health. Deliver information in small chunks and check parents understanding as you go
	Respond appropriately to verbal and non-verbal communications	Make sure there is sufficient time in the consultation to answer any questions that parents may have. Be sensitive to signs of distress in parents (e.g. arms folded) and children (fidgeting, clingy behaviour, avoiding eye contact). Respond by asking whether it is ok to continue, and whether there is any way you can make the conversation easier
Planning	Give time for families to process the news and its implications	Make sure families have contact details and an opportunity to follow-up any questions they may have in the following days

(Continued)

Table 6.1 (Continued)

Phase	Issues to consider	Application to the weight feedback situation
Follow-Up	Provide written information or a summary of your conversation	Supplement information given verbally with written information that explains anything that they might have missed during the consultation
	Give details of services and support organisations that may be able to help the family	Make sure you are aware of local services and places of support. Give parents good quality self-help materials to support self-directed efforts to change

should be limited to professional communication and documentation whereas less emotive synonyms (e.g. larger, bigger) should be used in direct communications with families [36]. In practice, the choice of what words to use may depend on the purpose of the conversation. It could be helpful to use medical terms such as 'obese' and 'overweight' in consultations where the purpose is to 'diagnose' the problem and highlight the serious health implications of the child's weight status as a means of building appropriate levels of concern. Nevertheless, continued use of such emotionally laden terminology is unlikely to be helpful beyond the initial diagnostic conversations. When it is useful to talk about a child's size as part of the process of supporting the family to make changes, it is more helpful to use euphemistic language (e.g. larger, heavier, bigger) as a way of preventing unnecessary distress and alienation.

As well as age and developmental stage, practitioners may also need to consider disease severity and the level of comorbidity. Generally, the more obese a child is, and the greater the impact that their excess weight has on their health, the more likely it is that the child will have to take a more active role in the management of the condition, even at younger ages. In such cases, practitioners will need to find age-appropriate ways to talk about excessive weight gain and its effects.

Addressing areas of particular sensitivity in weight-related conversations

Whilst using general principles of effective communication will certainly lead to more constructive conversations with families, there are a number of areas that can cause particular sensitivity or may get in the way of developing a family's commitment to behaviour change.

Addressing weight stigma and avoiding unintentional stigmatisation

Stigmatising attitudes and beliefs have their roots in misinformation, and the most effective way to address weight stigma is by educating parents and professionals about the myths and realities of the condition. As will be evident to readers of this book, the factors contributing to the development of obesity are enormously complex and research is still far from providing a complete understanding of the condition. In situations where there is an absence of certainty and the presence of complexity, most individuals – parents and professionals alike – are likely to fill in the gaps with their own beliefs or those present in wider society. Since the majority view of obesity is largely negative, this can lead to behaviour or attitudes that are unintentionally stig-matising. In discussions about child obesity, this most often manifests as explanations which grossly simplify the disorder, for example in explanations that emphasise single causes rather than complexity (e.g. 'it is all the fault of genetics/parents/schools'), in explanations or interventions that reflect the beliefs of the practitioner rather than expert consensus (e.g. focussing on *either* diet *or* activity to the exclusion of the other), or that focus inappropriately on one aspect of the obesogenic system to the exclusion of others (e.g. 'it is all the parent's fault'). In reality, families of children who become overweight are a very diverse group of people and there are an unlimited number of pathways that lead to the development of excess weight gain. Explanations or com-ments that ignore such heterogeneity in the ways that genes, environment and life-style interact to contribute to excessive weight gain are unhelpful as well as stigmatising. By working with families to understand the specific ways in which the family's lifestyle is contributing to a child's weight gain and avoiding the prescription of generalised advice, workers can avoid practices that are often experienced by families as stigmatis-ing, regardless of intent.

Addressing the role of genetics in the development of obesity

Obesity runs in families and it is very likely that overweight children will have one or more parents for whom weight is currently an issue, or has been in the past. Indeed, having an obese parent more than doubles the chances of a child being obese themselves, and if a child has two obese parents, they are 12 times more likely to be obese [37]. The tendency for obesity to run in families is primarily due to genetics, although the mechanisms by which genes exert their influence on bodyweight are multiple and complex [38]. It can be helpful for practitioners to have a convincing explanation of the role played by genes that helps parents under-stand that the genetic basis to the condition does not mean that obesity is inevita-ble. A helpful explanation may be that genes provide the potential for a child to gain weight more easily than others in environments that make it very easy for this to occur [39]. Most people in a population have genes that make it easy to gain weight and this is why over more than half of all adults and a third of all children are overweight. However, even if a child has genes that predispose them to gaining weight, becoming or staying overweight is not inevitable if they develop eating and activity habits that can protect them against future weight gain. It is the habits and behaviour (i.e. the family lifestyle) that parents teach their children which will determine whether a child's genes will result in them becoming or staying overweight.

Addressing feelings of blame, shame and guilt

The Oxford English Dictionary defines 'blame' as being 'responsible for a fault or wrong' [40]. Beliefs that parents are to blame for their child's weight status are based on the faulty assumptions that being overweight is somehow 'wrong' and that parents are the single most important factor in determining this outcome. As we have repeatedly seen in this book, a child becomes overweight as a result of a complex and poorly understood constellation of factors, many of which are beyond the parent's direct control. It can be helpful to point out that our children live in a cultural environment that is very toxic for their health and this is why so many parents are in the same position. Reassure those parents who feel guilty about not spotting the problem earlier that it is very diffi-cult to tell when a child has crossed the largely invisible boundary into an unhealthy weight status. In situations where strong feelings of blame or shame have the potential to disrupt the formation of an effective helping relationship, it is important to address this by directly reassuring parents that they are not to blame for the current situation, whilst simultaneously encouraging a belief that it is possible to take action to improve things for the future. Most psychologists agree that increasing feelings of blame and shame in parents rarely helps them to change difficult situations or unhealthy patterns of behaviour and may be counterproductive. It is useful to empathise with rather than dismiss any feelings of blame or shame that parents may express, whilst at the same time drawing their attention to the possibility of change and the options available to support this.

Addressing fears associated with psychological harm

Practitioners often report that parents are defensive during weight-management consultations. Generally, defensive behaviours arise when parents fear that a professional or procedure may cause harm or distress to their child. Fear of damaging self-esteem and causing an eating disorder is commonly cited by parents concerned about the impact of screening for obesity [11, 41]. As with other strong negative emotions, fear is best handled by enquiring about, and showing empathy for, the reasons behind the emotion. It can be helpful to share with parents that being overweight itself is a risk factor for the development of later eating problems. This is because children become more aware of negative attitudes and behaviours towards their size as they get older and may try to engage in unhealthy methods of losing weight to address this [4, 42–45]. It can also be helpful to reassure parents that most interventions to help children manage their weight are designed to improve the way children think and feel about their bodies, whatever their actual weight, and research shows that overweight children who take part in such programmes have less chance of developing an eating disorder than would be the case if they had been left to manage it without support [46]. Parents who have experienced eating disorders themselves, or in close family members, may be especially concerned about talking to children about their weight. Such parents may value the chance to explore their concerns with a psychologist with experience of working with families where weight and body image issues may mean that they have a more complex relationship to receiving support.

Beyond identification

Accurate and sensitively carried out identification of obesity is an important first step in helping families engage with the lengthy and effortful process of changing their lifestyle to promote the health of their children. However, research shows that only a small number of families are able to translate such information into sustainable action that results in clinically significant weight reduction. Therefore, an important part of the initial screening or identification conversation should involve linking families to resources that can help them make changes. This could be self-help information, or information about local services. Expert consensus guidance suggests that multi-component programmes combining dietary education, physical activity and behaviourally-based parenting support are likely to secure the best outcomes for children (e.g. [47]).

CASE STUDY

Mrs Jones brings her 4-year-old son, Jake, with her to a consultation with a Health Visitor to get some help about his poor sleeping patterns. The service has a policy of routinely checking children's height and weight during all consultations for the purposes of monitoring development.

The Health Visitor plots Jake's height and weight on a boy's BMI chart. After giving advice about improving Jake's sleeping patterns, she broaches the issue of Jake's weight status. In order to do this sensitively, the Health Visitor has directed Jake to go to the supervised play area so she can talk openly with his mum:

Health Visitor:	You noticed that we measured Jake's height and weight when you came into the centre today. I thought you might be interested in how he is getting on in terms of his growth. As well as looking at how tall he is, we are also interested in whether his height and weight are in proportion for his age. If you look at this chart here (the Health Visitor references the BMI chart on which she has worked out Jake's weight status), you will see that this is where Jake is today. This shaded area here (points to the blue shaded area indicating a healthy BMI status) represents the range where children's height and weight are in proportion, which means they are a healthy weight for their age. Jake is currently above this range and actually above this line here (refers to the line indicating the 98th percentile). Jake is above a healthy weight for his age and height and falls into the range that doctors would refer to as obesity. I don't know whether you had been concerned about Jake's weight. What do you think about this news?
Mrs Jones:	What do you mean? Are you saying my son is fat?
Health Visitor:	It sounds like this news might be a bit of a shock. It's not the sort of news that any parent likes to hear, especially when they may not have been expecting it. I am saying that at the moment Jake is carrying too much weight for his height and age and this is likely to lead to health problems if we can't do something about this. Look, this is a lot to take in; can I ask what your thoughts are about this?
Mrs Jones:	Honestly, it's a shock. I wasn't expecting to be told about this. Are you sure? Are you even allowed to tell me this without a doctor? Obese – I hate that word!
Health Visitor:	Sure, I understand. It's a really horrible word. This chart here is a very reliable measure and so I am 100% sure that your GP would say the same thing. You have probably heard lots on the news about the health problems associated with being overweight in childhood, and so it's now part of our role as health visitors to monitor this part of children's development. It is upsetting to find this out but the reason we want to let you know is that the earlier we catch it the more likely that we can do something about it. Would you have preferred not to know?
Mrs Jones:	No, I suppose not. I just feel so bad. He's no bigger than any of the other kids in his class. I just thought he was normal. I don't understand what I am doing wrong.
Health Visitor:	You are not doing anything wrong. Over half of all adults in the UK are overweight and over a third of children are overweight. Most parents can't tell when their kids are overweight and that's why we have to use these charts. Jake is a gorgeous, lively little boy. All we have to do is help you make a few changes to his eating and activity habits, and eventually he will grow into his weight and move towards this blue zone here.
Mrs Jones:	But we have a really healthy diet at home, we are not eating take-out every night.
Health Visitor:	I am sure you are not. It may take a while to figure out what is causing this. It is very, very unlikely to be anything medical. I am going to give you some leaflets about what Jake should be eating for his age and the amount of exercise he should be doing. Take these leaflets, have a read and try and work what might need to change. If you can't figure it out, don't worry, we can help with that. We have some really good groups on healthy eating here at the centre as well as access to a dietitian. We will continue to monitor his growth every 6 months, so that you can tell if he is moving in the right direction.

TAKE HOME MESSAGES

- Children's weight status is a sensitive topic for most parents. Practitioners working in this field should expect and be equipped to deal constructively with such sensitivities.
- There is a culture of avoidance when talking about child obesity. Parents wish to avoid their child being labelled and professionals fear upsetting or alienating parents. In both cases, the current and future health of the obese and overweight child is compromised.
- Many parents' sensitivities arise from wanting to protect their children from the harmful effects of weight stigma. Professionals can contribute to breaking down weight stigma by educating families about the complexity of factors leading to excessive weight gain and providing information that helps dispel unhelpful myths about the condition.
- Whilst most parents agree that childhood obesity is a serious issue, relatively few are able to correctly identify their own child's weight status, even if this might seem obvious to a health professional. This may explain why many community-based child weight management programmes struggle to recruit children into their services, even when located in areas where obesity has a high prevalence.

References

1 Gilman SL. *Fat: A cultural history of obesity*. Polity: Cambridge, 2008.
2 Puhl R, Latner J. Stigma, obesity and the health of the nations children. *Psychol Bull* 2007; **133**: 557–580.
3 Puhl R, Heuer C. The stigma of obesity: a review and update. *Obesity* 2009; **17**: 941–964.
4 Neumark-Sztainer D. Weight based teasing among adolescents: correlation with weight status and disordered eating behaviours. *Int J Obes Relat Metab Disord* 2002; **26**: 123–131.
5 Hayden-Wade HA, Stein RI, Ghaderi A, Saelens BE, Zabinski MF, Wifley DE. Prevalence, characteristics, and correlates of teasing experiences among overweight children vs non-overweight peers. *Obes Res* 2005; **13**: 1381–1392.
6 Puhl R, Luedicke J, Heuer C. Weight-based victimisation toward overweight and obese adolescents: observations and reactions of peers. *J Sch Health* 2011; **81**: 696–703.
7 Berry D, Colindres M, Vu MB. Latino caregivers' insights into childhood overweight management and relationships with their health care providers. *Hisp Health Care Int* 2009; **7**: 11–20.
8 Edmunds LD. Parents perceptions of health professionals responses when seeking help for their overweight children. *Fam Pract* 2005; **22**: 287–292.
9 Pagnini D, King L, Booth S, Wikenfeld R, Booth M. The weight of opinion on childhood obesity: recognising complexity and supporting collaborative action. *Int J Pediatr Obes* 2009; **4**: 233–241.
10 Turner KM, Salisbury C, Shield JPH. Parents' views and experiences of childhood obesity management in primary care: a qualitative study. *Fam Pract* 2012; **29**: 476–481.
11 O'Keefe M, Coat S. Consulting parents on childhood obesity and implications for medical student learning. *J Pediatr Child Health* 2009; **45**: 573–576.
12 Grimmet C, Croker H, Carnell S, Wardle J. Telling parents their child's weight status: psychological impact of a weight-screening programme. *Pediatrics* 2008; **122**: 682–688.
13 Stop Obesity Alliance. *Weigh-in: Talking to your children about weight and health*. http://www.stopobesityalliance.org/wp-content/themes/stopobesityalliance/pdfs/stopobesityalliance-weighin.pdf (accessed 6 April 2014).
14 Rietmeijer-Mentink M, Paulis WD, van Middelkoop M, Patrick JE, Bindels PJE, van der Wouden JC. Difference between parental perception and actual weight status of children: a systematic review. *Matern Child Nutr* 2013; **9**: 3–22.
15 Binkin N, Spinelli A, Baglio G, Lamberti A. What is common becomes normal: the effect of obesity prevalence on maternal perception. *Nutr Metab Cardiovasc Dis* 2013; **23**: 410–416.
16 Jones AR, Parkinson KN, Drewett RF, Hyland RM, Pearce MS, Adamson AJ, and the Gateshead Millennium Study core team. Parental perceptions of weight status in children: the Gateshead Millennium Study. *Int J Obes* 2011; **35**: 953–962.
17 Keller KL, Olsen A, Kuilema L, Meyermann K, van Belle C. Predictors of parental perceptions and concerns about child weight. *Appetite* 2013; **62**: 96–102.
18 Nihiser AJ, Lee SM, Wechsler H, McKenna M, Odom E, Reinold C, Thompson D, Grummer-Strawn L. BMI measurement in schools. *Pediatrics* 2009; **124**: 89–97.

19 Kubik MY, Fulkerson JA, Story M, Rieland G. Parents of elementary school students weigh in on height, weight, and body mass index. *J Sch Health* 2006; **76** (10): 496–501.

20 Johnson A, Ziolkowski GA. School-based body mass index screening programmes. *Nutr Today* 2006; **41**: 274–279.

21 Kalich KA, Chomitz V, Peterson KE, McGowan R, Houser RF, Must A. Comfort and utility of school-based weight screening: the student perspective. *BMC Pediatr* 2008; **8**: 9.

22 Kubik MY, Story M, Davey C. Obesity prevention in schools: current role and future practice of school nurses. *Prev Med* 2007; **44**: 504–507.

23 Routh K, Rao JN, Denley J. A simple, and potentially low-cost method for measuring the prevalence of childhood obesity. *Child Care Health Dev* 2006; **32**: 239–245.

24 Westwood M, Fayter D, Hartley S, Rithalia A, Butler G, Glasziou P, Bland M, Nixon J, Stirk L, Rudolf M. Childhood obesity: should primary school children be routinely screened? A systematic review and discussion of the evidence. *Arch Dis Child* 2007; **92**: 416–422.

25 Chomitz VR, Collins J, Kim J, Kramer E, McGowan R. Promoting healthy weight among elementary school children via a health report card approach. *Arch Pediatr Adolesc Med* 2003; **157**: 765–772.

26 West DS, Raczynski JM, Phillips MM, Bursac Z, Gauss CH, Montgomery BEE. Parental recognition of overweight in school-age children. *Obesity* 2008; **16**: 630–636.

27 Park MH, Falconer CL, Croker H, Saxena S, Kessel AS, Viner RM, Kinra S. Predictors of health-related behaviour change in parents of overweight children in England. *Prev Med* 2014; **62**: 20–24.

28 Falconer C, Park M, Skow A, Black J, Sovio U, Saxena S, Kessel A, Croker H, Morris S, Viner R, Kinra S. Scoping the impact of the national child measurement screening programme feedback on the child obesity pathway: study protocol. *BMC Public Health* 2012; **12**: 783.

29 Syrad H, Falconer C, Cooke L, Saxena S, Kessel AS, Viner R, Kinra S, Wardle J, Croker H. 'Health and happiness is more important than weight': a qualitative investigation of the views of parents receiving written feedback on their child's weight as part of the National Child Measurement Programme. *J Hum Nutr Diet* 2014; doi: 10.1111/jhn.12217.

30 Ikeda JP, Crawford PB, Woodward-Lopez G. BMI screening in schools: helpful or harmful. *Health Educ Res* 2006; **21**: 761–769.

31 The Health and Social Care Information Centre, Lifestyle Statistics. *National Child Measurement Program: England, 2011/12 school year*. The NHS Information Centre for Health and Social Care: Leeds, 2012.

32 Walker O, Strong M, Atchinson R, Saunders J, Abbott J. A qualitative study of primary care clinicians vies of treating childhood obesity. *BMC Fam Pract* 2007; **8**: 50–57.

33 Committee on Hospital Care. American Academy of Pediatrics. Family-centred care and the pediatricians role. *Pediatrics* 2003; **112** (3 Pt.1): 691–697.

34 Royal College of Nursing. *Breaking bad news: Supporting parents when they are told of their child's diagnosis*. http://www.rcn.org.uk/__data/assets/pdf_file/0006/545289/004471.pdf (accessed 18 March 2014).

35 Edvardsson K, Edvardsson D, Hornsten A. Raising issues about children's overweight – maternal and child health nurses experiences. *J Adv Nurs* 2009; **65**: 2542–2551.

36 Barlow SE. Expert committee recommendations regarding the prevention, assessment and treatment of child and adolescent overweight and obesity. *Pediatrics* 2007; **120** (Suppl 4): 164–192.

37 Whitaker KL, Jarvis MJ, Beeken RJ, Boniface D, Wardle J. Comparing maternal and paternal intergenerational transmission of obesity risk in a large population-based sample. *Am J Clin Nutr* 2010; **91**: 1560–1567.

38 Farooqi SI, O'Rahilly S. Genetic factors in human obesity. *Obes Rev* 2007; **8** (Suppl 1): 37–40.

39 Bray GA. Leptin and leptinomania. *The Lancet* 1996; **348** (9021): 140–141.

40 Oxford University Press. *Oxford English Dictionary*. Oxford University Press: Northamptonshire, 2010.

41 Eneli IU, Kalogiros ID, McDonald KA, Todem D. Parental preferences on addressing weight-related issues in children. *Clin Pediatr* 2007; **46**: 612–618.

42 Sim LA, Lebow J, Billings M. Eating disorders in adolescents with a history of obesity. *Pediatrics* 2013; **132** (4): e1–e5.

43 Stice E, Cameron RP, Killen JD, Hayward C, Taylor CB. Naturalistic weight-reduction efforts prospectively predict growth in relative weight and onset of obesity among female adolescents. *J Consult Clin Psychol* 1999; **6**: 967–974.

44 Fairburn CG, Cooper Z, Doll HA, Welch SL. Risk factors for anorexia nervosa: three integrated case control comparisons. *Arch Gen Psychiatry* 1999; **56**: 468–476.

45 Fairburn CG, Welch SL, Doll HA, Davies BA, O'Connor ME. Risk factors for bulimia nervosa: a community-based case control study. *Arch Gen Psychiatry* 1997; **54**: 509–517.

46 Epstein LH, Valoski A, Wing RR, McCurley J. Ten-year outcomes of behavioural family-based treatment for childhood obesity. *Health Psychol* 1994; **13**: 373–383.

47 National Institute for Health and Care Excellence. *Managing overweight and obesity among children and young people: Lifestyle weight management services: NICE public health guidance* **47**. http://www.nice.org.uk/nicemedia/live/14298/65523/65523.pdf (accessed 7 April 2014).

CHAPTER 7

Parenting strategies for healthy weight in childhood

Clare Collins, Tracy Burrows and Kerith Duncanson
Priority Research Centre in Physical Activity and Nutrition, Faculty of Health and Medicine, The University of Newcastle, Callaghan, Australia

Introduction

Preventing childhood obesity and achieving healthy growth and healthy weight in childhood are important ways to reduce the risk of adult obesity and the risk factors for chronic disease, including elevated blood levels of cholesterol, glucose and insulin. Childhood is a critical time during which healthy eating habits and food preferences are established. Even if a child maintains a healthy weight throughout the entire childhood period, they can still develop unhealthy eating habits that then track through to adulthood and increase the risk of adult obesity and associated chronic disease risk factors. Hence, although this chapter describes obesity prevention strategies and concepts, the focus will be on parenting practices for the establishment of healthy dietary patterns, eating habits and food preferences that are conducive to achieving healthy weight status throughout the lifecycle, and with consideration of cultural, societal and environmental influences.

The term 'healthy eating' is usually used in the context of nutritional quality of food and dietary intake of food groups. However, 'healthy eating' also encompasses the habits related to food and eating that could lower the risk of lifestyle-related chronic disease. For example, evidence suggests that sitting at a table to eat, having meal time routines and avoiding television (TV) viewing at meal times are equally as important in the development of healthful food-related behaviours as the nutritional value of foods served [1].

The role of parents and the techniques they use in the context of child feeding is paramount in determining child weight status and longer-term lifestyle-related chronic disease risk. Parents are the main influence on a child's dietary intake until the child goes to school. While parents continue to exert influences beyond this critical early childhood period, peers and significant others become increasingly influential. The eating habits and food preferences developed in this critical early life period evolve from their feeding environment, innate taste preferences [2] and their health and medical history. For example, it is possible that the trajectory for child dietary intake and preferences around food may be interrupted by major illness that impacts on appetite or digestive function.

For the purposes of this chapter, the term 'parenting' will be used to explain how a parent influences a child's behaviours and development [3]. Parenting style represents the

Early Years Nutrition and Healthy Weight, First Edition. Edited by Laura Stewart and Joyce Thompson.
© 2015 John Wiley & Sons, Ltd. Published 2015 by John Wiley & Sons, Ltd.

culmination of parental attitudes and beliefs towards child rearing and creating an emotional climate through which parental practices are expressed [4], including the quality of parent–child interactions. Parenting styles consist of two independent dimensions:

1 Demandingness or control, defined as the extent to which parents influence children by way of behaviour regulation, direction confrontation and supervision of the child's activities [4].

2 Responsiveness or nurturance, defined as the extent to which parents foster individuality and self-assertion by being attuned and supportive towards children's requests including supporting development of their independence and use of reasoned communication [5].

By cross-matching these two dimensions, four categories of parenting style have been defined:

1 Authoritative, characterised as being highly demanding of the child, but also highly responsive to their needs. This is typified by parental involvement, nurturance and expectations with monitoring of child behaviour.

2 Authoritarian (highly demanding, low responsiveness) characterised by restrictive, punitive and power-assertive parenting behaviours.

3 Indulgent or permissive (low demanding and high responsive) characterised by warmth and acceptance in conjunction with a lack of monitoring of child behaviour.

4 Uninvolved (low demanding, low responsive) characterised by little control, nurturance or involvement with the child [6].

While it is acknowledged that parenting style once established can be difficult to change, even with targeted interventions [7], it is important for health practitioners to understand how parenting style may impact on child dietary intake and child weight status. Authoritative parenting has been associated with increased fruit and vegetable availability and lower intake of energy-dense, nutrient-poor foods such as sweetened foods and drinks and salty snacks [8]. An authoritarian parenting style (highly demanding, but not very responsive) has been associated with higher body mass index and total fat mass [9] and with lower intake of fruit, juices and vegetables [10]. Surveys have revealed that approximately 40% of parents believe that restricting or forbidding a child's intake of foods high in fat and sugar is effective in decreasing their preferences for those foods, but this is not supported by epidemiological research [9]. A permissive parenting style has also been associated with child overweight [11] and with the dietary practices of drinking less milk and lower consumption of all nutrients except fat [8].

Some researchers have conceptualised a third dimension of 'structure', defined as the ways in which parents organise their child's environment to achieve their desired child-rearing goals, and that includes aspects of parent behaviour such as consistency, organisation and proactive strategies including providing opportunities and modelling of behaviours [12]. Structured households consist of an organised environment in which parents provide clear rules, set boundaries, provide support and guidance for following the rules, and these aspects are consistently enforced [12].

When parenting style is applied in a child-feeding context, more specific feeding styles have been described, which are a derivative of parenting style based on two dimensions related to the feeding context [13]. Responsiveness refers to how the parents encourage eating or the level of nurturance that parents use in directing their children's eating. Demandingness refers to how much the parent encourages eating or how demanding they are during the eating experience. Four types of child-feeding styles have been proposed to correspond to those from parenting style. The development

Box 7.1 Health practitioner reflection

Health practitioners can reflect on how the shift away from more authoritarian parenting styles dominant in past generations has influenced child feeding and child weight status. If parenting had become generally more authoritative over the past generation or two, this should have reflected positively on child weight status within the current generation. While positive parenting programmes are intended to develop parenting skills that are consistent with an authoritative parenting style, it is possible that the trend towards more child-centric parenting has gone beyond authoritative towards a more generally permissive parenting style, which is potentially detrimental in a child health context.

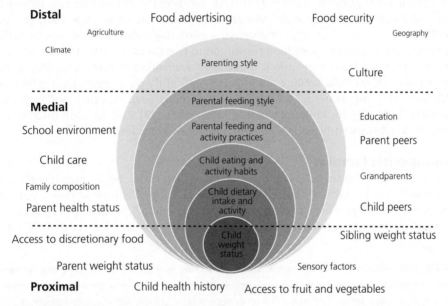

Figure 7.1 Spheres of influence on child's weight status.

of feeding styles or 'food parenting' provides a logical link between the more proximal and generalised parenting style and very specific child-feeding practices or behaviours exhibited by parents and measured by researchers (see Box 7.1).

Parenting practices are specific goal-directed parent actions or behaviours designed to influence children's behaviours [4]. Controlling 'food parenting' practices has been linked to lower self-regulation in eating [14] and higher child weight status [9].

The sphere of influence of parental, environmental, cultural, peer, child and other related factors on child weight status, including relationships, strength of influence and proximal versus distal level of influence [15], is shown in Figure 7.1.

The relative importance or strength of evidence around each factor is indicated by the size of the text, and the proximity of the influence to child weight status is shown by the positioning on the page from top (distal) to bottom (proximal). This diagram is intended to:

- provide practitioners with an overall concept relating to potential intervention points and
- assess the possible enablers and barriers that practitioners may experience when working at an individual, family or community level to achieve healthy weight.

Influence of parents on family eating styles, food and physical activity habits and sedentary behaviours

Childhood is a key timeframe for establishment of health behaviours [16]. To date, relatively few studies have explored development of eating-related health behaviours [14]. Children's eating behaviours are determined by some child-specific factors [17], some parent-specific factors [8] and the complex interactions between parents and their children (see Box 7.2) [18].

Parent-specific factors

Quantitative studies that have considered relationships between children's food choices and various environmental factors [19] have consistently shown that risk factors for poor childhood nutrition include poor maternal nutrition knowledge [20], parental television viewing, authoritarian or permissive parenting styles [21] and role modelling of energy-dense, nutrient-poor food consumption (see Box 7.2) [19]. Additionally, parents concern for disease prevention, home food availability, parental attitudes, beliefs and practices about child feeding, all impact significantly on a child's food intake and behaviours [19, 20]. Maternal self-efficacy has recently been reported by Campbell as positively impacting on children's eating behaviours [22] and an authoritative parenting style is consistently associated with optimal child feeding [23].

Child-specific factors

Factors that are intrinsic to the child that relate to their eating behaviours include temperament, neonatal history and feeding history [17, 24]. Taste preferences, appetite, growth and development are important related physiological factors [17] that vary substantially between children. In non-controlling, non-coercive conditions where

Box 7.2 Considerations for health professionals when working with parents on achieving healthy weight

1 Weight status may be interpreted differently depending on cultural and family background. For example, in some cultures, a higher weight is indicative of health and prosperity.
2 Food and eating are not only about weight, they also have important roles in socialisation and cultural inclusion.
3 Practitioners will benefit from focusing on achievement of healthy eating, physical activity and healthy weight, rather than focusing on obesity.
4 In the current food environment and the wider community environment, it is very challenging for parents to role model healthy lifestyle behaviours.
5 With increasingly challenging environmental influences, authoritative child-feeding practices need to be established early and maintained assertively by parents.
6 Parenting has changed considerably in the past one to two generations. One could now consider parenting to be a verb, an action word. It is possible that this shift towards child-centric parenting has impacted on child obesity.
7 Parents in individual families may be working in isolation to try to get children to be more active, but society reinforces and rewards sedentary behaviours.
8 Consistency between parents and other care givers increases the effectiveness of healthy lifestyle practices within families.
9 If parents are trying to role model physically active behaviours for their family, they need to be resilient, and expect to face barriers along the way. Practitioners who can empathise and pre-empt these barriers will help parents enormously in addressing barriers.
10 There are limitations and issues associated with measurement in most of the existing scales of parenting style and parenting practices that relate to food, physical activity and sedentary behaviours.

children have access to a variety of healthful foods, young children have the ability to self-regulate the amount of food and total energy consumed [14, 17].

These intrinsic child factors become influenced by and inextricably linked to environmental factors very early in a child's development [18]. Parents may negatively influence their children's dietary intakes and ability to self-regulate by applying excessive external control or failing to provide healthy options [9]. Completely banning highly palatable foods may promote the children's desire for them, causing dysregulation of energy intake, overeating and ultimately weight gain [9]. Based on limited observational studies, parental restriction of a child's dietary intake of highly palatable foods may be associated with child adiposity [9]. Conversely, food neophobia and food aversions can be minimised in an environment of positive role modelling and repeated exposure to these foods such that many disliked foods become tolerated and then eventually enjoyed over time (see Box 7.2) [25].

Parent–child interaction

The feeding relationship between parent and child (Figure 7.2) is established at birth and represents both a powerful connection and potential focus for 'power struggles' or control issues between parent and child [16]. The theory of the feeding relationship, first presented in 1992 by Satter [26], is that a parent is responsible for feeding a child appropriate foods at appropriate intervals, that is the 'what' and 'when' of the feeding relationship. The child is responsible for the ultimate decision regarding whether to consume the food or not and the portion they choose to eat of the food provided – the 'whether' and 'how much' of the feeding relationship. The 'parents provide, children

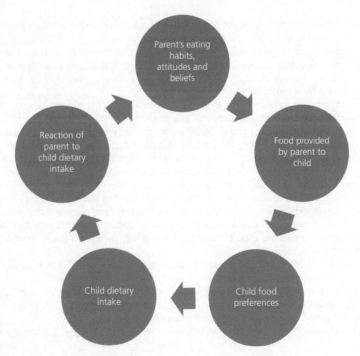

Figure 7.2 Parent/child feeding interaction relationships.

decide' theory is often used in nutrition programmes to assist with behavioural change and delineate the parent and child roles in the feeding relationship [27].

Parents do not treat all their children alike. Parenting practices are shaped by each child's characteristics, including sex, age, birth order, health and physical appearance [28]. Parental attempts to control and restrict children's food intakes become more intense with increasing child overweight, especially if the child is a girl [9].

Parent engagement

Parents are important agents of dietary behaviour development as the 'gate keepers' of their children's eating environments [18]. This is particularly true for young children, as a large proportion of their food is consumed within the home environment. Engagement of parents is therefore critical in any childhood nutrition intervention. The success of interventions aimed at changing parents lifestyle-related behaviours relies on promotion of the enablers and offsetting the barriers to parent engagement in health behaviour change, particularly those related to child feeding and childhood nutrition.

CASE STUDY

Emily is a 7-year-old girl who has been referred to a dietitian by a General Practitioner (GP) as her weight for age has continued to increase relative to height for age every year since she was 2 years old.

Weight: above 95th centile; height: 40th centile
Diet: limited variety of foods – less than 20 foods in diet

Health history: Emily was born 5 weeks premature with no known cause, after an uncomplicated pregnancy. She was breastfed from birth to 4 months of age, but had severe colic. She was introduced to solids at 3 months in an unsuccessful attempt to overcome colic. Emily did not transition through textures well and continued to eat predominantly pureed food and infant formula until she was 2 years old. She was underweight for height until 2 years of age, and so her parents were not inclined to increase food variety for fear of weight loss.

Emily started to eat larger amounts of food at 2 years of age, but her diet continued to be limited to one or two fruits (preferences changed), milk and yogurt (no lumps), sausages, potato and a wide range of breads, processed grains and discretionary foods. Emily and her brothers enjoy electronic games as none are particularly 'sporty' and all love reading and play musical instruments.

Parents: Mother works part time and tries hard to apply parenting principles she has learned at a community-based programme, where she identified her own parenting style as permissive. She finds it difficult to set boundaries and impose consequences. She does let Emily have choices and contribute to decision making. Mother is of European descent and food has always been a major family focus. Emily's grandmother cares for Emily and her two brothers (one older and one younger) after school and on some weekends when Emily's mother works. Father works full time and has a more authoritarian parenting style. He expects the children to eat their meals as a family, although he does eat in front of the TV in the evening.

Neither parent does any structured physical activity and as little incidental activity as possible. Dad loves his gadgets and time-saving devices.

Intervention: Initial consultations with mother and father to include an open, non-judgemental discussion including the following:
• Background information and open discussion of parental issues and concerns.
• Explanation of weight status and acknowledgement that parents are to be commended for taking action.

- Explanation of how a child's development is influenced by early life experiences such as progression of food textures, early childhood illness.
- Discussion relating to how parents' beliefs, background and culture impact on child development and weight status.
- Comparison of parents' attitudes to food and eating (may be different to each other).
- Discussion of family factors that may contribute to child weight status – role modelling of father, feeding style of mother, levels and type of restriction, pressure to eat, monitoring and perceived responsibility.
- Introduction of the 'parents provide, children decide' philosophy relating to parents providing appropriate portions of suitable foods and the child deciding whether and how much (from suitable amount provided) they will eat.
- Discussion of possible barriers to changing family food and activity environment, for example role of grandparents as carers

Following initial consultation, treatment options will be discussed. These could include family sessions including Mum, Dad (and siblings) and Emily, or a family-based group program if available. Either option will include a combination of information, practical demonstrations and 'homework' for the family members with all having a role to play, including grandmother.

Based on the information provided and discussions in the initial consultation/s, priority areas for family action would be developed, with goals established to commence the process of changing family food and activity environment.

In addition to face-to-face group or individual programmes, evidence-based resources such as DVDs, books or online programs could be recommended to the family.

Sample practitioner goals

Increase understanding of Emily's weight status in context of all influencing factors.
Provide a suite of choices for family action and assist family to prioritise their strategies.
Support and guide family in changing food and activity environment.
Facilitate a change process that is mutually positive for all family members.
Sample goals for parents to implement changes in family food and activity environment:

1 Provide up to two choices for meals and monitor portions.
2 Provide structure to meal and snack times, with maximum of one snack between each meal.
3 Increase range of foods using a sensory approach, working across the spectrum of colours and textures, within family meal times and 'practice sessions'.
4 Implement the 'parents provide, children decide' eating philosophy.
5 Include Emily in selection and preparation of meals at least twice a week, giving her two choices to select from.
6 Provide opportunities for active play.
7 Take Emily for a walk each day, including some time in a park for free play.
8 Eat family meals at the table with TV turned off.
9 Monitor physical activity and sedentary time and establish agreed limits for both.

Outcomes

- Increased awareness (without blame) of factors contributing to Emily's current weight status awareness of priority areas for change and agreement on course of action.
- Progressively improved family food and physical activity environment.
- Understanding, support and collaboration between key family members and significant others, including peers, grandmother, teachers, family friends and brothers.

Results

- Weight stability or slight weight decrease as height increases to achieve weight under 75th centile by age 10 years.
- Lifelong eating and activity habits established.
- Family eating and activity habits improved, minimising risk for all generations.

TAKE HOME MESSAGES

These issues will present additional challenges for practitioners when working with families towards achieving healthy weight

- Single parent families in which one parent is assuming full responsibility for child. This can result in parent being more permissive because it is difficult to manage food parenting alone.
- Separated families in which care of children is shared and each parent has different attitudes and beliefs around food parenting, or food is used as a bargaining tool.
- Families in which grandparents invest considerable time in caring for children but indulge children with food. The role of carer versus grandparent becomes blurred.
- Low general parental efficacy or parent self-efficacy.
- Food being used as a reward or punishment.
- Fussy eating (father) or restrictive eating (mother).
- Low availability of healthy food group choices.
- High availability and accessibility of energy-dense, nutrient-poor 'junk' foods.
- High visibility but low access (overt restriction) to energy-dense, nutrient-poor 'junk' foods.
- Pressure to eat 'You will finish your dinner'.
- Inappropriate use of discretionary foods as reward.
- Foods available outside designated meal/snack time.

List of options for parents to positively influence eating style/ habits

- Family meals together at table with television (TV) off.
- High availability of healthy foods in the home environment (and restriction of 'junk' discretionary foods without child being aware).
- Monitoring of child dietary intake relative to requirements.
- Appropriate use of energy-dense nutrient poor foods for celebrations/cultural or symbolic reasons.
- Role modelling healthy eating habits.
- Involvement of children in food preparation.
- Communication about food and nutrition with school/childcare.
- Increasing skills to minimise the impact of food marketing, for example turn the TV off.
- Understanding food labelling.
- Replacing use of food as a reward with non-food rewards.
- Accessing appropriate nutrition resources.
- Minimising the impact of fussy eating (father) and restrictive eating (mother).
- Minimising child eating alone or 'sneaky' eating.
- High availability and accessibility of core healthy foods.
- Minimising pressure to eat 'You will finish your dinner'.
- Minimising foods available outside designated meal/snack time.
- Positive feedback/praise for trying new foods or for healthy eating behaviours.

List of options for parents to positively influence physical activity habits and sedentary behaviours

- Family physical activity – 'families that play together, stay together'.
- Ensuring access to physical activity options – skate boards, skipping ropes, hula hoops, and trampolines.
- Understanding and assisting development of fundamental movement skills.
- Monitoring of child sedentary time.
- Role modelling healthy activity habits.
- Involving children in activity – walk together without stroller.
- Communication about activity and fundamental movement skills with school/childcare.
- Understanding child physical activity and sedentary behaviour guidelines.

How can a practitioner help families to change food and physical activity environment?

- Use a collaborative, whole-agency approach involving family, health professionals and significant others.
- Recognise mutual expertise between practitioner and parent, acknowledging that parents are trying their best and are capable of behavioural change.
- Match strategies, resources and support to level of readiness to change for each goal/area that parent wants to address.
- Recognise the importance of 'getting and keeping' or 'engaging' parents.
- Encourage strategies that establish authoritative parenting styles and 'normalise' parenting support.
- Target parenting skills to parent-cited concerns, for example overcoming fussy eating and how to increase food variety.
- Ensure parents have access to quality, culturally and linguistically appropriate resources related to healthy eating and good nutrition that are appropriate and user friendly.
- Respond in a timely manner to parental concerns.
- Minimise but understand potential feelings of isolation or victimisation and fear of being labelled a 'bad parent' or a failure.
- Increase awareness of consequences of behaviours to decrease risk of ambivalence or unwillingness to change own behaviours.
- Allow time between exposure and expected adoption of health behaviour change.

References

1 Dietz W, Robinson T. Overweight children and adolescents. *N Engl J Med* 2005; **352** (20): 2100–9.
2 Skinner J, Carruth B, Wendy B, *et al*. Children's food preferences; a longitudinal analysis. *J Am Diet Assoc* 2002; **102**: 1638–47.
3 Bornstein MH. *Handbook of Parenting*. Lawrence Erlbaum Associates: Mahwah, 2002.
4 Darling N, Steinberg L. Parenting style as context: an integrative model. *Psychol Bull* 1993; **113**: 487–96.
5 Baumrind D. Current patterns of parental authority. *Dev Psychol* 1971; **4** (1 Pt.2): 1–103.
6 Maccoby E, Martin J. Socialization in the context of the family: parent-child interaction. In: Hetherington EM (ed), *Handbook of Child Psychology: Socialization, Personality and Social Development*. Wiley: New York, 1983, pp. 1–101.
7 Burrows T, Warren J, Collins C. The impact of a child obesity treatment intervention on parent child-feeding practices. *Int J Pediatr Obes* 2010; **5** (1): 43–50.
8 Patrick H, Nicklas T, Hughes S, *et al*. The benefits of authoritative feeding style: caregiver feeding styles and children's food consumption patterns. *Appetite* 2005; **44**: 243–9.
9 Fisher JO, Birch LL. Restricting access to foods and children's eating. *Appetite* 1999; **32**: 405–19.
10 Weber-Cullen K, Baranowski T, Rittenberry L, *et al*. Socioenvironmental influences on children's fruit, juice and vegetable consumption as reported by parents: reliability and validity of measures. *Public Health Nutr* 2000; **3** (3): 345–56.
11 Wake M, Nicholson JM, Hardy P, *et al*. Preschooler obesity and parenting styles of mothers and fathers: Australian National Population Study. *Pediatrics* 2007; **120** (6): 1520–7.
12 Hughes SO, O'Connor TM, Power TG. Parenting and children's eating patterns: examining control in a broader context. *Int J Child Adoles Health* 2008; **1**: 323–30.
13 Hughes SO, Power TG, Fisher JO, *et al*. Revisiting a neglected construct: parenting styles in a child-feeding context. *Appetite* 2005; **44**: 83–92.
14 Birch LL, Fisher JO, Davison KK. Learning to overeat: maternal use of restrictive feeding practices promotes girls' eating in the absence of hunger. *Am J Clin Nutr* 2003; **78**: 215–20.
15 Egger G, Binns A, Rossner S. *Lifestyle Medicine: Managing Diseases of Lifestyle in the 21st Century*, 2nd edition. McGraw Hill: Sydney, 2011.
16 Rosenthal M, Crowley A, Curry L. Promoting child development and behavioural health: family child care providers' perspectives. *J Pediatr Health Care* 2009; **23** (5): 289–97.

17 Birch LL, Fisher JO. Development of eating behaviours among children and adolescents. *Pediatrics* 1998; **101** (3): 539–49.

18 Daniels L, Magarey A, Battistutta D, *et al*. The NOURISH randomised control trial: positive feeding practices and food preferences in early childhood – a primary prevention program for childhood obesity. *BMC Public Health* 2009; **9**: 387.

19 Campbell KJ, Crawford DA, Ball K. Family food environment and dietary behaviors likely to promote fatness in 5–6 year-old children. *Int J Obes* 2006; **30** (8): 1272–80.

20 Vereecken CA, Keukelier E, Maes L. Influence of mother's educational level on food parenting practices and food habits of young children. *Appetite* 2004; **43**: 93–103.

21 Golan M, Crow S. Targeting parents exclusively in the treatment of childhood obesity: long-term results. *Obes Res* 2004; **12**: 357–61.

22 Campbell K, Hesketh K, Silverii A, *et al*. Maternal self-efficacy regarding children's eating and sedentary behaviours in the early years: associations with children's food intake and sedentary behaviours. *Int J Paediatr Obes* 2010; **5**: 501–8.

23 Duke RE, Bryson S, Hammer LD, *et al*. The relationship between parental factors at infancy and parent-reported control over children's eating at age 7. *Appetite* 2004; **43** (3): 247–52.

24 Birch L. Development of food preferences. *Annu Rev Nutr* 1999; **19**: 41–62.

25 Benton D. Role of parents in the determination of the food preferences of children and the development of obesity. *Int J Obes Relat Metab Disord* 2004; **28** (7): 858–69.

26 Satter E. Eating competence: nutrition education with the Satter Eating Competence Model. *J Nutr Educ Behav* 2007; **39**: 189–94.

27 Burrows T, Warren JM, Baur LA, *et al*. Impact of a child obesity intervention on dietary intake and behaviours. *Int J Obes* 2008; **32** (10): 1481–8.

28 Brann LS, Skinner JD. More controlling child-feeding practices are found among parents of boys with an average body mass index compared with parents of boys with a high body mass index. *J Am Diet Assoc* 2005; **105** (9): 1411–16.

CHAPTER 8

Pre-school prevention interventions

Pinki Sahota

School of Health and Wellbeing, Leeds Beckett University, Leeds, UK

Introduction

Childhood obesity is a growing problem internationally [1, 2]. High rates of childhood obesity are prevalent in pre-school children, and it is estimated that 9.5% of children in the UK [3] and 21% of children in the USA [4] are already obese at school entry. Data from epidemiological studies indicate that this epidemic begins in early childhood [5–7] with evidence emerging about the impact of obesity on early health. A recent study found that metabolic markers of high cholesterol, blood pressure and abnormal glucose metabolism were already present at the age of 9 years [8]. Other studies have shown that children as young as 3–8 years old already have early vascular lesions [9]. Furthermore, obesity once established is known to track into adulthood and contributes to obesity-related co-morbidities such as heart disease, diabetes, certain cancers and osteoarthritis [10]. The early years of childhood is a critically important time for establishing healthy eating behaviours and motor skills [11, 12]. As diet and physical activity are associated risk factors, it is recommended that efforts to prevent obesity should focus on early childhood so that habits which are normally established at this early age [13, 14] can be positively influenced [15].

Parents are ultimately responsible for their children's development, but with many parents in full or part-time employment, child care providers may also play an important role by providing opportunities for children to be active and develop healthy eating habits and by acting as positive role models [16]. Current evidence suggests that behaviours that contribute to obesity can be positively impacted in a range of settings and provides important insights into the most effective strategies for promoting healthy weight from early childhood [17]. Child care settings provide many opportunities to promote healthy eating and physical activity behaviours among pre-school-aged children.

This chapter will examine the current evidence-base and highlight effective strategies and interventions for parents and carers with the home and early years' settings for the prevention of childhood obesity. Key messages related to establishing healthy diet, physical activity and sedentary behaviours will be presented. Finally an example of a government initiative from an international perspective will be presented as an illustration of good practice.

Research has demonstrated consistent associations between caregiver behaviour and child weight status throughout development [15]. Hesketh and Campbell [18]

Early Years Nutrition and Healthy Weight, First Edition. Edited by Laura Stewart and Joyce Thompson.
© 2015 John Wiley & Sons, Ltd. Published 2015 by John Wiley & Sons, Ltd.

concluded that 'parents are receptive to and capable of some behavioural changes that may promote healthy weight in their young children' (p.337), however interventions aimed at parents should focus not only on knowledge but also on the associated skills and competencies.

Family approach

It is suggested that children learn behaviours through observation and participating in joint activities and therefore parental and carer role modelling presents an ideal opportunity to promote positive behaviours. Research shows similarities in many aspects of mothers and daughters intake including beverage consumption, consumption of fruits and vegetables, and fat, mineral and vitamin intake. These findings reflect that a number of factors such as the types of foods that the mother prefers and consequently offers the child, the exposure and accessibility of these foods and the opportunity of eating together with parents at mealtimes are influential in promoting healthy eating behaviour. Parents and childcare providers should act as positive role models for children, through their own choices on healthy eating and physical activity [19].

Adults should be encouraged to sit with children and eat the same foods, thereby modelling the consumption of healthy foods [20], which in turn encourages children to eat the same foods [21]. Furthermore, it has been found that families who consistently have family mealtimes are less likely to have overweight children [22]; however, the social context of eating together must not be undervalued. Eating with others also reinforces healthy eating through activities such as sitting down and eating slowly which are associated with mindful eating thereby reducing the risk of overconsumption.

Availability and accessibility of food

Parents and carers also play a vital role in facilitating the development of healthy eating behaviours through the provision of healthy foods. The availability of healthy food increases exposure of such foods to the child and consequently greater likelihood of eating them. Additionally on a practical level for younger children, this food also needs to be accessible. Therefore cutting up fruits and vegetables as finger foods and offering them as snacks, is one way to promote consumption of such foods [19].

The feeding strategies that parents and carers adopt may inadvertently have a negative effect on their child's eating habits. One of the strategies that parents use in restricting foods they consider to be 'bad' and to encourage foods considered to be 'good' is using a preferred food as a reward for eating the less desired food. For example 'eat your vegetables and then you can have your dessert'. Recent research suggests that these strategies are counter-productive and often result in the child having a preference for the restricted food, that is the dessert. Studies indicate that restricting access to foods increased the preference for and consumption of those foods when they were no longer restricted. Furthermore restriction of food has been linked to increased fat intake and increased eating in the absence of hunger in girls. Strategies such as 'eat up' or 'clear your plate' have resulted in increasing a child's energy intake, increasing the fat content of the child's diet, reducing intake of fruits and vegetables, increasing the time a child spends eating and increasing the degree of child fatness [23].

Responsive feeding

More importantly by employing the aforementioned strategies, parents are encouraging their child to override their internal cues of hunger and fullness. There is clear evidence that young children have the ability to self-regulate their intake. Although energy intake may vary from meal to meal, consumption over a 24 hour period is more consistent [24].

Parent or carer control over all decisions related to children's food intake, including the amount eaten is shown to reduce the child's ability to self-regulate energy intake [25] and an increased risk of overweight in pre-school-aged children [26]. Furthermore, offering larger portions can also override the self-regulation mechanism with larger portions encouraging the child to overeat [27]. Therefore, parents and carers should be encouraged to follow responsive feeding practices by allowing children to determine how much they eat which in turn will reinforce internal cues for hunger and satiety and consequently result in self-regulation of energy intake (see Chapter 7).

Signals toddlers may use to indicate they have had enough food:

- Saying 'no'
- Keeping their mouth shut when food is offered
- Turning their head away from food being offered
- Pushing away a spoon, bowl or plate containing food
- Holding food in their mouth and refusing to swallow it
- Spitting food out repeatedly
- Crying, shouting or screaming
- Gagging or retching

Healthy eating

Parents and carers knowledge of what constitutes a healthy diet is a prerequisite for establishing healthy eating practices, and research shows that parents' nutrition knowledge is positively related to healthier eating behaviours in children [19]. However, research findings highlight that there is misunderstanding about what constitutes a healthy diet amongst many parents of young children. There is over concern about the lack of fruit and vegetables in their child's diet with no consideration of the concept that a healthy diet comprises of a variety of foods and food groups in balanced amounts [28].

In the absence of specific healthy eating guidelines for pre-school-aged children, it is suggested that the national guidelines based on models such as the Eatwell Plate in the UK [29], the Dietary Guidelines for Americans (DGA) for children aged 2 years and over [30] and the Australian Dietary Guidelines [31] should be used as a basis.

Most healthy eating models are based on the recommended principle that a healthy diet should comprise of a variety of food and drink from different food groups which should be consumed in different amounts. One example is the Eat Well Plate model shown which illustrates the food groups and the proportions that comprise a healthy balanced diet (Figure 8.1).

Surveys of dietary intake in pre-school-aged children indicate that many are not following the recommended healthy eating guidance. Surveys report consumption of high levels of energy-dense foods and low intakes of fruit and vegetables [32, 33] resulting in high energy intakes that contribute to the risk of overweight and obesity [34]. Of further concern is that such patterns are being established early and therefore foundations are being established for these eating patterns for later life. Table 8.1 below shows recommendations for a healthy balanced diet for pre-school-aged children.

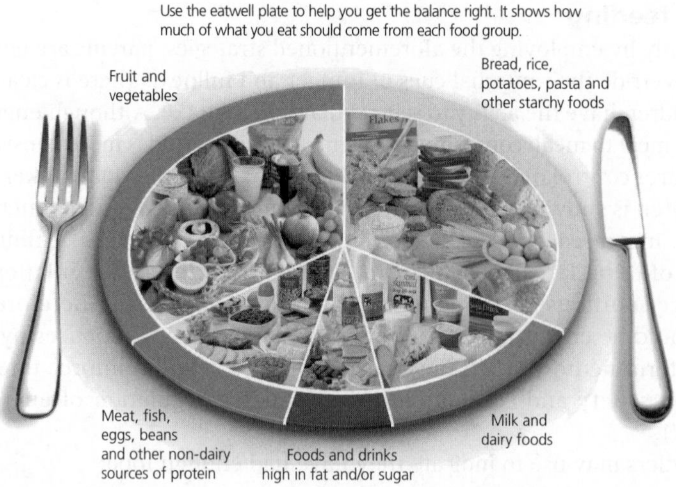

Use the eatwell plate to help you get the balance right. It shows how much of what you eat should come from each food group.

Fruit and vegetables

Bread, rice, potatoes, pasta and other starchy foods

Meat, fish, eggs, beans and other non-dairy sources of protein

Foods and drinks high in fat and/or sugar

Milk and dairy foods

Figure 8.1 The eatwell plate. Reproduced with permission from Public Health England. © Public Health England.

Table 8.1 Healthy eating in toddlers.

Food groups	Recommendations
Bread, cereals, potatoes	At least one food from this group at each meal and at most snack times
Fruit and vegetables	At each meal, aim for five small servings or tastes each day
Milk, cheese and yogurt	Serve three times per day
Meat, fish and alternatives	Once or twice per day for meat- and fish-eating children
	Two to three times a day for those who only eat eggs, pulses
Foods high in fat, sugar and salt	Can be offered in addition to four food groups but not instead of
Drinks	Six to eight drinks (100–150 ml) per day from breaker or cup; milk and water are best; fruit juice well diluted

Based on 10 steps for a healthy toddler (www.infantandtoddlerforum.org).

Energy-dense foods

To prevent the development of overweight and obesity in their child, parents and carers should consider some specific aspects in relation to energy intake. Energy-dense foods (cakes, biscuits, savoury snacks, crisp type snacks and confectionary) should be made less available within the home and child care settings. Whole grains, fruit and vegetables are good sources of complex carbohydrates, fibre, vitamins and minerals, and due to their fibre and water content, they are lower in energy density and thereby help to promote satiety and fullness for longer. Children should be encouraged to establish preferences for foods with lower energy density and higher nutrient content such as fruit and vegetables, which result in improved nutrient intakes, lower energy consumption without reducing the size of the meal [35] and consequently reduce the risk of obesity.

Drinks

Sugar-sweetened drinks such as fizzy and fruit drinks are commonly consumed by children and are energy dense and nutrient poor. There is strong evidence of the links between the intake of sugar-sweetened drinks and excess weight gain in young children

[36]. Furthermore, early introduction of these drinks establishes preferences for such beverages in later life [23]. However, recent surveys show that more than half of pre-school-aged children consume one or more servings of sweetened drinks per day [32, 33] which contribute 60 kcal/day to the diets of 2- to 3-year olds [37]. Although consumption of 100% fruit juices is not linked to overweight, higher energy intakes have been found in children who consumed these juices. Therefore, limiting 100% fruit juice to no more than one serving per day in a cup has been suggested for pre-school-aged children [38]. Water has been recommended as an alternative to sugar-sweetened drinks and fruit juice in an attempt to reduce total energy intake [39].

Portion sizes

There is much confusion amongst parents about appropriate portion sizes with few guidelines or resources available to assist in improving this understanding. By late pre-school age, children become more responsive to external cues than to their innate ability to self-regulate intake. When presented with larger portions, older children will consume the larger quantities compared to younger children who demonstrate better self-regulation [40]. An increase in portion sizes is considered to be an important contributing factor to the obesity epidemic. Studies show a parallel between increasing portion sizes and rising obesity rates for children and adults. The increase in portion size is particularly evident for energy-dense foods such as snack foods and servings in fast-food restaurants. Therefore, educating parents about age-appropriate portion sizes is considered key in promoting healthy eating and alleviating anxieties related to insufficient intake. However, it must be emphasised that requirements vary from time to time and child to child, and recommended portion sizes should be used as a guide to how much should be presented on the plate. Other strategies may include avoiding the use of adult size plates for younger children which encourages inappropriately large portions. Recent helpful resources on portion sizes have been produced within the UK by The Infant and Toddler Forum (www.infantandtoddlerforum.org) and The Carolyn Walker Trust (www.cwt.org.uk) which can be accessed via the respective websites.

Regular meals

Energy intake can also be regulated by encouraging parents and carers to establish structured eating patterns rather than allowing children to 'graze' throughout the day. By establishing a routine and offering meals at set intervals and limiting eating occasions to three meals and two snacks per day, the overall energy intake can be controlled. The meals should comprise ideally of two courses and thereby provide a wide range of nutrients. Pre-school-aged children are often unable to obtain sufficient nutrients required through three meals and therefore need additional nutritious snacks of food combinations from the first four food groups such as fruit and vegetables, small sandwich, breadsticks or crackers with cubes of cheese and celery sticks. Meal and snack times should be spaced at regular intervals throughout the day in order to prevent feelings of excess hunger and tendency to overeat.

Physical activity and sedentary behaviour

Inactivity in the early years is a key contributor to childhood obesity and impaired physical, cognitive and emotional development. A systematic review [41] of the impact of sedentary behaviour found that under-4-year-olds spend up to 84% of their waking hours being inactive by sitting in a buggy, being restrained in a car seat or chair or in front of a screen. Associations were evident between sedentary behaviour and adiposity, bone and skeletal health, motor skills, psychosocial health (such as self-esteem), and cognitive development and cardiometabolic health. In particular, there was a strong correlation between television (TV) viewing and adiposity and decreased scores on measures of psychosocial health and motor skill development. Another study which tracked 1314 young children found a connection between TV viewing hours and increased waist circumferences. Pre-school-aged children who watched TV more than 2 hours a day had increased waist circumferences of 7.6 mm by the age of 10 years [42].

Another influence of TV viewing is the impact on dietary intake. Children are not only inactive, but they are also exposed to advertisements for unhealthy foods. A recent European study of 15, 144 children found that those who had their meals in front of the TV also developed a preference for foods high in fat and sugar [43]. Furthermore, the distraction of watching TV whilst eating may lead to reduced awareness of appetite and recognition of internal cues for satiety resulting in overconsumption.

There is also concern that habits learnt in the early years may shape activity levels in later life. Guidelines on physical activity published by UK Health Departments [44] acknowledge the problem, but make no recommendations about upper limits for sedentary behaviour, stating only that carers should minimise the amount of the time under-fives spend this way. They recommend that pre-school-aged children who are walking should be physically active for 3 hours a day. Most UK pre-school-aged children currently spend 120–150 minutes a day in physical activity, so achieving this guideline would mean adding another 30–60 minutes/day. Pre-school-aged children are unlikely to be able to sustain long periods of activity; therefore, several short bursts throughout the day are recommended to achieve the recommendation through activities such as playing in the park, walking up stairs, bouncing on a trampoline, dancing, running and walking to nursery. The Australian Government [45] and the latest Canadian guidelines [46], which have been shaped by the systematic review, are discussed in Chapter 5.

> Recommendations for parents and carers for the prevention of childhood obesity in pre-school-aged children:
> - Model a healthy lifestyle
> - Take a whole family approach
> - Encourage responsive feeding
> - Limit availability and accessibility of energy-dense food in the home
> - Limit consumption of sweet drinks and increase consumption of water
> - Encourage acceptance of healthy foods – including fruit and vegetables
> - Ensure portion sizes are appropriate for age
> - Establish meal routines
> - Encourage 180 minutes physical activity per day
> - Limit sedentary activities including screen time to less than 1 hour/day

Obesity prevention and early years settings

Early years settings play an important role by providing opportunities for children to be active and develop healthy eating habits. Recent guidance recommends all nurseries and child care facilities to prioritise prevention of excess weight gain and improve children's diet and activity levels [16]. The following actions are suggested:

- Establishing mealtime routines.
- Ensure that children eat regular, healthy meals in a pleasant, sociable environment, free from other distractions (such as TV).
- Children should be supervised at mealtimes and ideally staff should eat with children.
- All action aimed at preventing excess weight gain, improving diet (and reducing energy intake) and increasing activity levels in children should involve parents and carers.
- Minimise sedentary activities during play time and provide regular opportunities for enjoyable active play and structured physical activity sessions.
- Implement guidance on food procurement and healthy catering, for example UK Department for Education, Children's Food Trust and Caroline Walker Trust guidance.

Existing evidence from the USA indicates the following may be successful strategies for promoting healthy eating and physical activity in child care settings, although it is not clear which combinations of specific strategies are effective for reducing childhood obesity:

- integrating opportunities for physical activity into the classroom curriculum;
- modifying food service practices;
- providing classroom based nutrition education and
- engaging parents through educational newsletters or activities.

Few interventions have been evaluated to determine their impact on child weight status within child care settings. Table 8.2 shows details of some promising programmes. All interventions are multi-component interventions that are designed to promote healthy diet and physical activity behaviours through a variety of mechanisms ranging from carer and parent involvement, building community capacity or modifications in the organisational policy and environmental aspects of child care settings.

Table 8.2 Promising childhood obesity prevention programmes in the child care setting.

Programme title		
Prevention through Activity in Kindergarten Trial (PAKT) (age: 4–5 years) Roth et al. (2010) [47], Germany	Aim to increase young children's level of physical activity, improve motor skills and decrease health-risk factors and media use. Also to equip parents and children to continue activities after the programme had ended	Positive outcomes in terms of decrease in body mass index (BMI) and increased activity
Romp & Chomp (age: 0–5 years) de Silva-Sanigorski et al. (2010) [48], Victoria, Australia	Romp & Chomp aims to build and sustain local community capacity to promote healthy eating and active play in early childhood care and education settings. Activities include professional development for early years staff, support for new policy development and governance structures as well as social marketing strands	Decrease in BMI in those reported as overweight or obese compared to control group. Effective in establishing partnerships and collaborative working among key players
Nutrition and Physical Activity Self-Assessment for Child Care (part of Steps to a Healthier Arizona) (in pre-school-aged children) Drummond et al. (2009) [49] Arizona, USA	Pilot intervention, designed to assist childcare providers in implementing changes to organisational practices, policy and environment to promote healthy eating and physical activity behaviours in young children. Delivered by 'Steps' coordinator via seven workshops. Evaluation based on assessment of best practice in settings.	Improved practice in childcare settings reported and 'ripple effect' extending impact beyond original scope. Sustainable and transferable. No findings on obesity/overweight outcome measures
'Hip-Hop to Health Jr.' program Fitzgibbon et al. (2005) [50], Chicago USA	Three weekly classroom lessons, classroom-based physical activity and weekly parent newsletters for 14 weeks. classroom-based physical activities were teacher-led and were provided three times per week for 20 minutes	Smaller increases in BMI in intervention group at 1 and 2 year follow-up Reduced calories from saturated fat in intervention group

CASE STUDY

In the USA, a national study of Head Start programmes in 2008 showed that most had instituted key practices to prevent obesity.

Head Start is a federal child development programme that serves low-income children aged 3–5 years with the overall goal to increase the school readiness of these children. To achieve this goal, Head Start provides a comprehensive range of services, including nutrition services. A number of federal regulations for Head Start programmes address the promotion of healthy eating and physical activity. The regulations help to ensure that:
- Parents receive guidance on nutrition and physical activity.
- Facilities participate in the Child and Adult Care Food Programme which includes:
  o reimbursement provided to child care centres and family childcare providers for up to either two meals and one snack or one meal and two snacks daily;
  o meals and snacks include a minimum number of age-appropriate servings from four food categories: fluid milk; vegetables, fruit or 100% juice; grains or bread; and meat or meat alternatives.
- Meals and snacks provide one-third to one-half of the daily nutritional needs of children in part-day and full-day programmes, respectively.
- Staff model healthy eating behaviours and attitudes for children.
- Facilities provide opportunities for outdoor and indoor active play, and adequate space.
- Facilities provide equipment to promote active play and opportunities to develop gross and fine motor skills.

Results of a randomised-controlled evaluation in 12 Head Start centres serving primarily African-American pre-school-aged children showed that those enrolled at centres assigned to the intervention had smaller increases in BMI compared with control children at 1-year and 2-year follow-up assessments. Children enrolled in the intervention were found to consume fewer calories from saturated fat compared to control children at 1-year follow-up. However, intake of total fat and dietary fibre per 1000 calories, physical activity frequency and intensity, and hours of daily TV viewing were similar among children enrolled in the intervention and control children at both 1-year and 2-year follow-up assessments.

TAKE HOME MESSAGES

- Parental and carer practices associated with child eating and physical activity habits include:
  o feeding styles,
  o the degree to which parents and carers provide a healthy environment such as access to healthy foods and physical activity facilities,
  o role modelling of healthy behaviours
  o nutrition knowledge [15].
- Pre-school-aged child care settings should provide opportunities for promoting healthy behaviours.

References

1 World Health Organization. Obesity: preventing and managing the global epidemic. Report of a WHO consultation. *World Health Organ Tech Rep Ser*. 2000; **894**: 1–253.
2 Wang Y, Monteiro C, Popkin BM. Trends of obesity and underweight in older children and adolescents in the United States, Brazil, China and Russia. *Am J Clin Nutr* 2002; **75** (6): 971–977.
3 Health and Social Care Information Centre, Lifestyle Statistics/Department of Health. *Health and Social Care Information Centre, Lifestyle Statistics*. http://www.hscic.gov.uk/catalogue/PUB09283/nati-chil-meas-prog-eng-2011-2012-rep.pdf (accessed 18 September 2014).
4 Ogden C, Carroll M, Curtin L, *et al*. Prevalence of high body mass index in US children and adolescents, 2007–2008. *JAMA* 2010; **303** (3): 242–249.
5 Singhal A, Fewtrell M, Cole TJ, *et al*. Low nutrient intake and early growth for later insulin resistance in adolescents born preterm. *Lancet* 2003; **361**: 1089–1097.

6 Baird J, Fisher D, Lucas P, *et al.* Being big or growing fast: systematic review of size and growth in infancy and later obesity. *BMJ* 2005; **331**: 929–931.

7 Stettler N, Stallings VA, Troxel AB, *et al.* Weight gain in the first week of life and overweight in adulthood – a cohort study of European American subjects fed infant formula. *Circulation* 2005; **111**: 1897–1903.

8 Gardner DS, Hosking J, Metcalf BS, *et al.* Contribution of early weight gain to childhood overweight and metabolic health: a longitudinal study (EarlyBird 36). *Pediatrics* 2009; **123** (1): 67–73.

9 Speiser PW, Rudolf MC, Anhalt H, *et al.* Childhood obesity. *J Clin Endocrinol Metab* 2005; **90** (3): 1871–1887.

10 Oude-Luttikhuis H, Baur L, Jansen H, *et al.* Interventions for treating obesity in children. *Cochrane Databases Syst Rev* 2009; **1**: CD001872.

11 Skinner J, Carruth B, Bounds W, *et al.* Children's food preferences: a longitudinal analysis. *J Am Diet Assoc* 2002; **102** (11): 1638–1647.

12 Hagan J, Shaw J, Duncan P, eds. *Bright Futures: Guidelines for Health Supervision of Infants, Children, and Adolescents.* 3rd ed. American Academy of Pediatrics: Elk Grove Village, 2008.

13 Birch L, Fisher J. Development of eating behaviours among children and adolescents. *Pediatrics* 1998; **101**: 539–549.

14 Trost SG, Sirard JR, Dowda M, *et al.* Physical activity in overweight and non-overweight preschool children. *Int J Obes* 2003; **27**: 834–839.

15 Skouteris H, McCabe M, Swinburn B, *et al.* Parental influence and obesity prevention in pre-schoolers: a systematic review of interventions. *Obes Rev* 2011; **12**: 315–328.

16 Nation Health Service. *Obesity: The Prevention, Identification, Assessment and Management of Overweight and Obesity in Adults and Children.* National Institute for Health and Clinical Excellence: London, 2006.

17 National Health Service. *Management of Obesity: A National Clinical Guideline 115.* Scottish Intercollegiate Guidelines Network: Edinburgh, 2010.

18 Hesketh KD, Campbell KJ. Interventions to prevent obesity in 0–5 year olds: an updated systematic review of the literature. *Obesity* 2010; **18** (1): 27–35.

19 Davison KK, Birch LL. Childhood overweight: a contextual model and recommendations for future research. *Obes Rev* 2001; **2**: 159–171.

20 Nicklas TA, Baranowski T, Baranowski JC, *et al.* Family and child-care provider influences on preschool children's fruit, juice, and vegetable consumption. *Nutr Rev* 2001; **59** (7): 224–235.

21 Addessi E, Galloway AT, Visalberghi E, *et al.* Specific social influences on the acceptance of novel foods in 2–5-year-old children. *Appetite* 2005; **45** (3): 264–271.

22 Taveras EM, Rifas-Shiman SL, Berkey CS, *et al.* Family dinner and adolescent overweight. *Obes Res* 2005; **13** (5): 900–906.

23 Birch LL. Development of food preferences. *Annu Rev Nutr* 1999; **19**: 41–62.

24 Birch LL, Johnson SL, Andresen G, *et al.* The variability of young children's energy intake. *N Engl J Med* 1991; **324** (4): 232–238.

25 Faith MS, Scanlon KS, Birch LL, *et al.* Parent-child feeding strategies and their relationships to child eating and weight status. *Obes Res* 2004; **2** (11): 1711–1722.

26 Rhee KE, Lumeng JC, Appugliese DP, *et al.* Parenting styles and overweight status in first grade. *Pediatrics* 2006; **117** (6): 2047–2054.

27 Fisher JO, Liu Y, Birch LL, *et al.* Effects of portion size and energy density on young children's intake at a meal. *Am J Clin Nutr* 2007; **86** (1): 174–179.

28 Wordley J, Sahota P, Borkoles E, *et al.* HELP, an obesity prevention intervention for parents of toddlers: barriers influencing behaviour change. *Obes Facts* 2009; **2** (Suppl 2): 66–67.

29 Public Health England. *The Eat Well Plate.* https://www.gov.uk/government/uploads/system/uploads/attachment_data/file/237282/Eatwell_plate_booklet.pdf (accessed October 2013).

30 USDA and HHS. *Dietary Guidelines for Americans* (2010). http://www.healthierus.gov/dietaryguidelines (accessed September 2013).

31 Australian Government National Health and Medical Research Council Department of Health and Ageing. *Healthy Eating for Children: Teach Your Child Healthy Habits for a Healthy Life.* http://www.eatforhealth.gov.au/sites/default/files/files/the_guidelines/n55f_children_brochure.pdf (accessed February 2014).

32 Department of Health. *National Diet and Nutrition Survey: Headline Results from Years 1, 2 and 3 (Combined) of the Rolling Programme 2008/09–2010/11.* http://webarchive.nationalarchives.gov.uk/20130402145952/http://transparency.dh.gov.uk/2012/07/25/ndns-3-years-report/ (accessed October 2013).

33 Fox MK, Condon E, Briefel RR, *et al*. Food consumption patterns of young preschoolers: are they starting off on the right path? *J Am Diet Assoc* 2010; **110** (12): 52–59.

34 Bradlee ML, Singer MR, Qureshi MM, *et al*. Food group intake and central obesity among children and adolescents in the third national health and nutrition examination survey (NHANES III). *Public Health Nutr* 2010; **13** (6): 797–805.

35 Leahy KE, Birch LL, Rolls BJ. Reducing the energy density of multiple meals decreases the energy intake of preschool-age children. *Am J Clin Nutr* 2008; **88** (6): 1459–1468.

36 Hu FB, Malik VS. Sugar-sweetened beverages and risk of obesity and type 2 diabetes: epidemiologic evidence. *Physiol Behav* 2010; **100** (1): 47–54.

37 Reedy J, Krebs-Smith SM. Dietary sources of energy, solid fats, and added sugars among children and adolescents in the United States. *J Am Diet Assoc* 2010; **110** (10): 1477–1484.

38 Baker SS, Cochran WJ, Greer FR, *et al*. The use and misuse of fruit juice in pediatrics. *Pediatrics* 2001; **107** (5): 1210–1213.

39 Wang YC, Ludwig DS, Sonneville K, *et al*. Impact of change in sweetened caloric beverage consumption on energy intake among children and adolescents. *Arch Pediatr Adolesc Med* 2009; **163** (4): 336–343.

40 Rolls BJ, Roe LS, Meengs JS. Larger portion sizes lead to a sustained increase in energy intake over 2 days. *J Am Diet Assoc* 2006; **106**: 543–549.

41 LeBlanc A, Spence JC, Carson V, *et al*. Systematic review of sedentary behaviour and health indicators in the early years (aged 0–4 years). *Appl Physiol Nutr Metab* 2012; **37**: 753–772.

42 Fitzpatrick C, Pagani LS, Barnett TA. Early childhood television viewing predicts explosive leg strength and waist circumference by middle childhood. *Int J Behav Nut Phys Act* 2012; **9** (87): 1–6.

43 Lissner L, Lanfer A, Gwozdz W, *et al*. Television habits in relation to overweight, diet and taste preferences in European children: the IDEFICS study. *Eur J Epidemiol* 2012; **27** (9): 705–715.

44 Department of Health. *UK Physical Activity Guidelines*. https://www.gov.uk/government/publications/uk-physical-activity-guidelines (accessed 7 April 2014).

45 Department of Health. *Get Up & Grow: Healthy Eating and Physical Activity for Early Childhood – Directors/Coordinators.* www.health.gov.au/internet/main/publishing.nsf/Content/phd-gug-directorscoord (accessed 7 April 2014).

46 Tremblay M, Leblanc AG, Janssen I, *et al*. Canadian sedentary behaviour guidelines for children and youth. *Appl Physiol Nutr Metab* 2011; **36**: 59–64.

47 Roth K, Mauer S, Obinger M, *et al*. Prevention through Activity in Kindergarten Trial (PAKT): a cluster randomised controlled trial to assess the effects of an activity intervention in preschool children. *BMC Public Health* 2010; **10** (410): 1–10.

48 de Silva-Sanigorski AM, Bell AC, Kremer P, *et al*. Reducing obesity in early childhood: results from Romp & Chomp, an Australian community-wide intervention program. *Am J Clin Nutr* 2010; **91** (4): 831–840.

49 Drummond RL, Staten LK, Sanford MR, *et al*. A pebble in the pond: the ripple effect of an obesity prevention intervention targeting the child care environment. *Health Promot Pract* 2009; **10** (2): 156–167.

50 Fitzgibbon M, Stolley M, Van Horn L, *et al*. Two-year follow-up results for Hip-Hop to Health Jr.: A randomized controlled trial for overweight prevention in preschool minority children. *J Pediatr* 2005; **146** (5): 618–625.

CHAPTER 9

Contribution of food provision in primary schools to the prevention of childhood obesity

Ethan A. Bergman

Department of Nutrition, Exercise, and Health Sciences, College of Education and Professional Studies, Academy of Nutrition and Dietetics, Central Washington University, Ellensburg, USA

Introduction

Prevention of obesity and maintaining optimum weight during childhood is important to improve the quality of life during childhood and beyond. Obesity is a multifactorial problem that includes community, school, families, physical activity and diet as well as components that are not as controllable such as genetics. This chapter does not discuss genetic factors but will include a brief overview of the types of programmes that are currently in place that address a healthful environment in the primary school setting. A brief mention of the types of programmes that are aimed at family support and community support is also included. The chapter also includes currently available healthful lifestyle initiatives that may be used in many settings. Whereas this chapter is devoted to prevention of obesity, the real issue that many countries face is promoting healthful eating and providing opportunities for adequate physical activity. Healthful eating includes consumption of the right amount of calories and nutrients through the foods available. As a consequence, this chapter will include the continuum of nutrition from undernutrition where the child consumes too few calories or too few nutrients. It will also include over consumption of calories, above the amount needed for daily needs. A US governmental department that seeks to promote a healthful environment in schools is the United States Department of Agriculture (USDA).

The United States Department of Agriculture

The USDA oversees the National School Lunch Program (NSLP), which is designed to provide meals to students who may not otherwise have access to a complete meal during the school day [1]. A primary goal of the NSLP has always been to level the field of success for school children of varying backgrounds by providing foods necessary for proper growth and development [2]. Students in the USA who do not participate in the NSLP bring their lunch from home. Insufficient nutritious foods in the proper proportions, or 'undernutrition', and the over consumption of some nutrients, or 'overnutrition', are major concerns for the health of youth for reasons pertaining to short- and long-term health, wellness, growth and success. There are two inter-related problems

Early Years Nutrition and Healthy Weight, First Edition. Edited by Laura Stewart and Joyce Thompson.
© 2015 John Wiley & Sons, Ltd. Published 2015 by John Wiley & Sons, Ltd.

that at first glance seem to be unrelated. In the year 2011, in the USA, 20.6% of households with children were food insecure [3]. Coincidently, the results from the 2007 to 2008 National Health and Nutrition Examination Survey (NHANES) indicate that an estimated 19.6% of children of ages 6–11 years are also overweight in the USA ([4]). Both undernutrition and overnutrition bear a heavy burden on the health of US children and children around the world. The NSLP is one way the USDA works to improve the integrity of child nutrition in the USA. Many countries have school meal–feeding programmes in place to help support physical and mental development, including the World Food Program (WFP).

The WFP provides meals to around 22 million children in 60 countries, often in the very remote and needy areas. For over 50 years, the WFP has been offering their services to help provide good nutrition to those needing it most. Today, the WFP is the largest provider of school meals in the world. The WFP often works in tandem with the governments to develop a quality and sustainable school-feeding programme [5].

Undernutrition can lead to serious health consequences in children. The quality and quantity of food that children consume contributes to both their ability to be academically successful as well as to their long-term health outcomes. It has been observed that children who are inadequately nourished are more likely to have delays in cognitive development [6, 7]. In addition, children who are undernourished may suffer from adverse behavioural and mental health problems [8]. Although the term 'malnutrition' has typically referred to the effects of undernutrition, it can also be used to describe overnutrition.

A state of overnutrition can occur when one or more nutrients are consumed in excess of what is required for normal development, growth and metabolism. Consumption of the nutrients fat and sugar in excessive amounts contributes to overweight, obesity and negative health outcomes. Health complications stemming from overnutrition include hypercholesterolaemia and hypertension, which in turn can contribute to chronic cardiovascular disease, type 2 diabetes and metabolic syndrome [9]. Furthermore, research suggests eating excessive fat and sugar and whether one perceives their own weight as healthy or not can have negative effects on mental health and learning [10, 11]. According to Francis and Stevenson [11], the hippocampus is impaired in people with diets high in fat and sugar, resulting in impaired memory function. In an analysis of a recent Youth Risk Behavior Survey, US children who identified themselves as being overweight were more likely to have been identified as having poor academic performance compared to those who identified themselves as having a normal weight [12]. As more evidence becomes available that school-aged children are at risk of developing academic-, behaviour- and health-related issues associated with over- and undernutrition, schools have become a target for improving the food served to and consumed by children.

School-feeding programmes are opportune places to address nutrition-related concerns

School-feeding programs throughout the world and the NSLP meals in the USA are opportune places to address the nutrition-related health concerns that plague children, and it is important those meals meet the nutritional needs of students. Since the inception of the NSLP in the 1940s, policies have been enacted to improve the quality of meals served in schools [2]. In 2011, 31 million children ate NSLP lunch each school day [1].

Because of the numbers of students who consume NSLP lunch daily, experts in the field of health and nutrition believe that school meals are advantageous places to address malnutrition-related health issues facing US children. The US Academy of Nutrition and Dietetics has published position papers that state continued importance of support for the government sponsored NSLP to fight malnutrition in American children and also calls for those meals to meet Dietary Guidelines for Americans [13]. The Academy of Nutrition and Dietetics Position paper on Local Support for Nutrition Integrity in schools states that schools and communities have a shared responsibility to provide students with access to high quality, affordable, nutritious foods and beverages [14].

The USDA has implemented a system of ensuring that students who need meals at school would either be free of cost or offered at a reduced cost, based on their families' average income compared to the poverty level. Any child attending a school that participates in NSLP may purchase a meal. Children from families with incomes at or below 130% of the poverty level are eligible for free meals. Reduced price meals are available for students from families with incomes between 130 and 185% of the poverty level. Children from families with incomes greater than 185% of the poverty level pay full price, and the price of the meal reflects a degree of subsidisation. For the 2012–2013 school year, 130% of the poverty level was $29, 965 for a family of four [1].

In order to assess the ability of meals served at school to meet the needs of children, the USDA sponsors the School Nutrition Dietary Assessment (SNDA) studies. The first SNDA study in 1991–1992 found that school lunches were high in fat and saturated fat compared to the recommended levels of the Dietary Guidelines for Americans [15]. The results of SNDA-I led to the implementation of the School Meals Initiative for Healthy Children (SMI) [14]. SMI required that schools offer meals that provide less than or equal to 30% of total energy from fat and less than 10% of total energy from saturated fat, while at the same time providing adequate levels of the target nutrients: calories, protein, calcium, vitamin A and vitamin C. Table 9.1 shows the SMI Guidelines for the Traditional Food-Based Menu Planning Method which was used in the four schools included in the current study. SNDA-II was conducted in the school year 1998–1999. It showed that schools had reduced fat and saturated fat levels in meals served, but school meals were still high in fat and saturated fat when compared to the standards established by SMI [15]. SNDA-III was reported most recently for data collected during the 2004–2005 school year.

SNDA-III analysed school meal quality based on the SMI nutrient standards, the Dietary Guidelines for Americans 2005 and the Dietary Reference Intakes (DRIs), which recommend nutrient intake levels needed for individuals to achieve a healthful diet and prevent disease [15]. Data were collected from district food service directors and their staff, school food service managers, principals, students and their parents in a nationally representative sample of 398 schools within 130 districts that offer federally subsidised school meals [15].

The results of SNDA-III show that more than 85% of schools offered reimbursable lunches that met the SMI standards for each of the key target nutrients: protein, vitamin A, vitamin C, calcium and iron [16]. When compared to the standards for energy, it was found that 61% of middle schools and 77% of high schools offered lunches that provided less energy than SMI standards require, while lunches offered in 40% of elementary schools provided less energy than required [17]. Most schools offered lunches that exceeded SMI standards for energy from fat and saturated fat: 81% of schools exceeded the standard for fat and 72% for saturated fat [17]. Only 6% of schools offered lunches that met all of the SMI standards. Sodium levels exceeded the recommendation at

Table 9.1 School Meals Initiative (SMI) for healthy children guidelines.

Minimum nutrient and calorie levels for school lunches

Traditional food-based menu planning approaches (School week averages)

	Minimum requirements	
Nutrients and energy allowances	**Group iii**	**Group iv**
	Grades k–3	**Grades 4–12**
	Ages 5–8	**Ages 9 and older**
Energy allowances (calories)	633	785
Total fat (as a % of actual total food energy)	<30%*,†	<30%†
Saturated fat (as a % of actual total food energy)	<10%*,‡	<10%‡
RDA for protein (g)	9	15
RDA for calcium (mg)	267	370
RDA for iron (mg)	3.3	4.2
RDA for Vitamin A (RE)	200	285
RDA for Vitamin C (mg)	15	17

*The Dietary Guidelines recommend that after 2 years of age, 'children should gradually adopt a diet that, by about 5 years of age, contains no more than 30% of calories from fat'.
†Not to exceed 30% over a school week.
‡Less than 10% over a school week.

almost all schools and very few lunches met the recommendation for fibre [16, 17]. SNDA-III showed that school meals typically provided appropriate amounts of protein, vitamin A, vitamin C, calcium and iron, but calories are sometimes underserved, and fat, saturated fat and sodium are often overserved to students.

Lunches brought from home

Not all students eat school-prepared meals. This is especially true worldwide where many school systems do not have a school-based feeding programme. Some students bring packed lunches brought from home (LBFH) or return home to eat their mid-day meal. Very few studies in the USA give insight into the nutritional quality of lunches the children bring from home compared to NSLP meals.

When specific foods were assessed in a smaller subsample ($n = 2314$ on day 1 of survey and $n = 666$ on day 2 through parent-assisted recall for elementary students) as part of SNDA-III, analysis did compare the dietary intake of NSLP participants and non-participants [15]. Nearly all NSLP lunch menus (96%) that were studied included one or more vegetable option in addition to any vegetables that were part of entrees. NSLP participants were more likely to consume vegetables than non-participants whose lunches were brought from home [15]. Similar findings showed that nearly all school lunch menus (94%) included fruit and NSLP participants were more likely to eat fruit at lunch than non-participants [15]. School lunch menus almost always (99%) offered flavoured milk which was usually low fat or skim, and NSLP participants were almost four times more likely than non-participants to drink milk at lunch (75 vs. 19%) [15].

When the daily energy intakes of a NSLP participant samples were compared to a matched sample of non-participants, it was found that elementary and high school students who participated in NSLP consumed an average of 130 kcal more than non-participants [15]. In elementary schools there were no significant differences in the adequacy of the usual intakes of vitamin A, vitamin B6, vitamin C, folate, thiamine, magnesium and phosphorous between NSLP participants and non-participants [15]. The percentage of energy from fat and saturated fat was comparable between NSLP participants and non-participants. NSLP participants had a significantly greater mean intake of fibre than non-participants across elementary, middle and high schools [15].

Earlier research into LBFH in the USA largely contrasts the results of SNDA-III. Rainville [18] found that the LBFH and NSLP meals had roughly the same number of calories. However, LBFH had more calories from fat and saturated fat. Rainville's study indicated that in LBFH fat and saturated fat provided 33% of the total calories in the meal. In comparison, fat and saturated fat accounted for only 29% of the calories in NSLP meals [18]. Unlike SNDA-III, Rainville found NSLP meals had significantly more protein as well as more of the vitamins A, B6, B12, D, folate, thiamine, and minerals, zinc, calcium and iron than LBFH. The LBFH had significantly more fat, sugar, carbohydrates and vitamin C. Both Rainville and SNDA-III agree that NSLP meals contain more fibre than LBFH as well as larger quantities of fruit and vegetables.

A recent study by Johnson, Bednar, Kwon, and Gustof [19] compared the LBFH meals of elementary students to USDA NSLP standards. The study was based on the standards used for analyses on the reimbursable school lunch requirements for elementary school (K-6). These requirements are designed to meet Dietary Guidelines for Americans and provide one-third of the daily Recommended Dietary Allowance for calories, protein, vitamins A and C, calcium and iron [19]. This study found that LBFH had fewer calories, less vitamin A, less calcium, less iron and less fibre than recommended in NSLP standards [19]. LBFH were in excess of nutrient requirement for protein, vitamin C and sodium, all of which were statistically significant ($p < 0.001$) [19]. Aside from specific nutrients, meals were also compared based on their food components.

The menu components of LBFH and NSLP meals were recently investigated and compared [19]. The researchers examined LBFH and NSLP lunches of second-grade students for the presence or absence of each of the following: vegetable, fruit, dairy item, high fat or high sugar snack, a fruit beverage other than water or 100% fruit juice. Only 45.3% of LBFH in the sample had fruit and 13.2% had a vegetable compared to NSLP meals where 75.9% contained fruit and 29.1% contained a vegetable. NSLP meals were significantly more likely to have a dairy component such as milk or yogurt. Analysis revealed that LBFH had significantly more high fat containing foods and more high sugar snacks and drinks than NSLP lunches [19]. Results suggest that NSLP meals contain more food components that are nutrient dense such as fruit, vegetable and dairy than LBFH. As evidence continues to reveal that children eat fewer servings of fruits and vegetables than recommended for optimal growth and development, it is important that children's lunches, LBFH or NSLP, provide healthy options.

The evidence that many LBFH are of low nutritional quality has come to the attention of health professionals and approximately 35% of students bring LBFH [18–20]. Johnston et al. [20] suggest an intervention for parents sending LBFH that includes suggesting the kinds of foods that would improve nutrient quality. This intervention would include focusing on fruit and vegetables which could be readily available in the home. In addition it is suggested that positively reinforcing students for making healthy food choices in LBFH could also serve as an area of intervention

[20]. Rainville [18] suggests advertising the superior quality and convenience of the NSLP to discourage bringing LBFH.

Based on the research studies to date, the nutritional quality of LBFH is uncertain. This could be a result of the variety of methods used to address the content of LBFH since they vary considerably. More research is needed to clarify the nutritional value of LBFH.

Initiatives to improve the school environment

Healthier US Schools Challenge

One example of a school-based programme is the Healthier US School Challenge (HUSSC). In addition to implementing more strict standards for target nutrients in school meals served to students through NSLP, USDA has developed a voluntary programme for schools to implement in an effort to address school-related activities that can contribute to wellness. The HUSSC encourages schools to promote healthy lifestyles by encouraging participation in NSLP. HUSSC also encourages serving more whole grains, and fruit and vegetables during meals as well as enacting a curriculum that includes nutrition education, physical education and wellness policies that promote healthy eating and exercise behaviours [20]. There are four levels of distinction: bronze, silver, gold and gold in distinction awards which can be earned by a school along with a monetary award. There are specific menu requirements for each award level for NSLP meals (Table 9.2). These include serving foods that meet current standards but also have less added sugar, fat and sodium [21]. Schools participating in HUSSC also make efforts to increase students' physical activity and focus on school-wide wellness standards and goals summarised in Table 9.3 [21].

Table 9.2 HUSSC Guidelines 2011–2012: food groups.

HUSSC requirement	Vegetables	Cooked dry beans or peas	Fruits	Whole grains	Milk
For all HUSSC-awarded schools	Offer a different vegetable every day of the week. Minimum serving: ¼ cup. Of these five servings, three must be dark green or orange	A serving of cooked dry beans or peas must be offered each week. Minimum serving: ¼ cup	Different fruit must be offered weekly. Minimum serving: ¼ cup/ serving	Incorporate whole-grain products, focusing on variety in the type of products and 'whole grain' listed as the first ingredient	Only offer low fat (1%) or fat free (skimmed) milk)
Silver level specification			Bronze and silver: one day per week	Bronze and silver: three times per week	
Gold level specification			Gold and gold in distinction: two days per week	One serving per day	

Table 9.3 HUSSC Guidelines 2011–2012: menu, food, and school health policies and practices.

HUSSC requirement	Menu practices	Competitive foods criteria	School health policies and practices
For all HUSSC-awarded schools	Every child should be able to select a reimbursable meal that meets the Challenge criteria. Menu items planned for the Challenge should be selected routinely by the students	Applies to all foods sold or served outside the school meals programmes; a la carte, vending, snack bar, school store	Fundraising, nutrition education, physical activity and wellness policy should all support a wellness environment and provide consistent messages
Silver level specification		Bronze and silver: applies during meals in all food service areas	
Gold level specification		Gold and gold in distinction: applies throughout the school day, throughout the school campus	

Initiatives to improve the family and community environment: Kids Eat Right

Family plays a huge role in developing a child's food environment. Kids Eat Right is a programme that works towards enhancing the family environment, to make it more healthy in many ways, including food and activity. Kids Eat Right is a joint initiative from the US Academy of Nutrition and Dietetics and Academy of Nutrition and Dietetics Foundation. This initiative supports US government efforts to help stop childhood obesity.

There are two parts to the Kids Eat Right programme. Firstly, there are parts that are aimed at the general public to help families make good decisions about food selection and physical activity. Secondly, there are parts of the programme that are focused on nutrition professionals, Registered Dietitians and Nutritionists, and Dietetic Technicians, who are well trained to provide consultation with the public related to helping families make wise choices.

The goals of the programme revolve around educating all levels of the community including parents, families, community and national policy makers about the importance of quality nutrition in childhood obesity prevention.

Kids Eat Right has three main objectives:
1 EDUCATE children, families, communities and policy makers on the importance of high-quality, nutritional foods in childhood obesity prevention efforts.
2 ADVOCATE on behalf of a quality-nutrition approach to promote growth and development.
3 DEMONSTRATE the food and nutrition expertise of registered dietitians through educational programming and advocacy [22].

The Kids Eat Right website (www.eatright.org/kids/) provides resources for the public and professionals to include in menu selection and activities that are helpful in preventing childhood obesity. For example, there are sections that include ideas for families to use in the kitchen, including methods of food preparation and ways to include children in food preparation. The website also offers insights into selection of ingredients for recipes, including ways to improve the nutrient intake of children. Sections on what to eat and how to incorporate healthy foods into a diet to improve the diet balance are also found. Kids Eat Right includes ways to increase family and individual activity.

Community-based programmes

When children are not in school or with their families, they are in the surrounding community. This could mean they are in the geographical location near their place of residence. However, community also takes on other meanings, such as race, ethnicity and socio-economic status [23]. The community, in all of its meanings, can have an enormous impact on the health of children. Having a community support system is a valuable resource to help implement programmes, organise social events that offer healthy food and activity options, and educate and encourage people to adopt and maintain healthy living parameters. Community programmes, such as farmer's markets may play key roles in supporting local business, while providing healthy options to community members [23].

Organisations within the community may promote good nutrition and physical activity such as organised group walking to school endeavours. The safety of the community is also an important part of community organisations, helping to motivate families and children to be physically active [24].

Additional programmes that may increase activity include providing play groups within safe play areas or building safe bike paths that may be used by community members. Building and maintaining community gymnasiums and other supervised physical activities help maintain opportunities for physical activity. The community can also influence the media to promote programmes that enhance physical activity such as healthy harvest fairs and physical activity events such as races. All of these community related activities work towards promoting healthy childhood weight [24].

TAKE HOME MESSAGES

- Helping school-aged children maintain healthy weights and avoid obesity requires a multifactorial approach that includes families, communities and schools.
- Schools are an ideal venue for incorporating approaches which include good nutrition and opportunities for vigorous and plentiful physical activity.
- Successful programmes provide children the opportunity for a well-balanced diet with adequate calories as well as the opportunity for plentiful and vigorous physical activity.

References

1 United States Department of Agriculture. *National School Lunch Program: Program Fact Sheet*. http://www.fns.usda.gov/cnd/lunch/AboutLunch/NSLPFactSheet.pdf (accessed 10 November 2014).
2 Stitzel K. Child nutrition programs legislation. *Top Clin Nutr* 2004; **19** (1): 9–19.
3 Coleman-Jensen A, Nord M, Andrews M, Carlson S. *Household Food Security in the United States in 2011*. *USDA*. http://www.ers.usda.gov/media/884525/err141.pdf (accessed 5 April 2014).
4 Ogden CL, Carroll MD, Curtin LR, Lamb MM, Flegal KM. Prevalence of high body mass index in US children and adolescents, 2007–2008. *JAMA* 2010; **303** (3): 242–249.
5 World Food Programme. *School Meals*. http://www.wfp.org/school-meals?icn=homepage-school-meals&ici=ourwork-link (accessed 7 April 2014).

6 Kapil U, Bhavna AA. Adverse effects of poor micronutrient status during childhood and adolescence. *Nutr Rev* 2002; **60** (5): 84–90.
7 Otero GA, Aguirre DM, Porcayo R, Fernández T. Psychological and electroencephalographic study in school children with iron deficiency. *Int J Neurosci* 1999; **99**: 113–121.
8 Juby C, Meyer EE. Child nutrition policies and recommendations. *J Soc Work* 2011; **11**: 375–386.
9 Freedman DS, Zuguo M, Srinivasan SR, Berenson GS, Dietz WH. Cardiovascular risk factors and excess adiposity among overweight children and adolescents: the Bogalusa Heart Study. *J Pediatr* 2007; **150** (1): 12–17.
10 Economos CD, Irish-Hauser S. Community interventions: a brief overview and their application to the obesity epidemic. *J Law Med Ethics* 2007; **35**: 131–137.
11 Francis HM, Stevenson RJ. Higher reported saturated fat and refined sugar intake is associated with reduced hippocampal-dependent memory and sensitivity to interoceptive signals. *Behav Neurosci* 2011; **125** (6): 943–955.
12 Florin TA, Shults J, Stettler N. Perception of overweight is associated with poor academic performance in US adolescents. *J Sch Health* 2011; **81** (11): 663–670.
13 Stang J, Bayerl CT, American Dietetic Association. Position of the American Dietetic Association: child and adolescent nutrition assistance programs. *J Am Diet Assoc* 2010; **110** (5): 791–799.
14 Bergman EA. Position of the Academy of Nutrition and Dietetics: local support for nutrition integrity in schools. *J Acad Nutr Diet* 2010; **110** (8): 122–131.
15 Gordon A, Cohen R, Crepinsek M, Fox M, Hall J, Zeidman E. The third School Nutrition Dietary Assessment Study: background and study design. *J Am Diet Assoc* 2009; **109** (Suppl 2): 20–30.
16 Story M. The third School Nutrition Dietary Assessment Study: findings and policy implications for improving the health of US children. *J Am Diet Assoc* 2009; **109** (Suppl 2): 7–13.
17 Gordon A, Crepinsek M, Briefel R, Clark M, Fox M. The third School Nutrition Dietary Assessment Study: summary and implications. *J Am Diet Assoc* 2009; **109** (Suppl 2): 129–135.
18 Rainville AJ. Nutritional quality of reimbursable school lunches compared to lunches brought from home in elementary school is two Southeastern Michigan districts. *J Child Nutr Manag* 2001; **25** (1): 13–18.
19 Johnson CM, Bednar C, Kwon J, Gustof A. Comparison of nutrient content and cost of home-packed lunches to reimbursable school lunch nutrient standards and prices. *J Child Nutr Manag* 2009; **33** (2): 1–8.
20 Johnston CA, Moreno JP, El-Mubasher A, Woehler D. School lunches and lunches brought from home: a comparative analysis. *Childhood Obes* 2012; **8** (4): 364–368.
21 United States Department of Agriculture: Food and Nutrition Service. *Healthy US Schools Challenge: Application Criteria.* http://www.fns.usda.gov/sites/default/files/2012criteria_chart.pdf (accessed 10 November 2014).
22 Kids Eat Right. *About Kids Eat Right.* http://www.eatright.org/kids/content.aspx?id=6442459728 (accessed 7 April 2014).
23 Economos CD, Hyatt RR, Goldberg JP, Must A, Naumova EN, Collins JJ, Nelson ME. A community intervention reduces BMI z-score in children: Shape Up Somerville first year results. *Obesity* 2007; **15** (5): 1325–1336.
24 Tucker P, Irwin JD, Bouck LM, He M, Pollett G. Preventing paediatric obesity; recommendations from a community-based qualitative investigation. *Obes Rev* 2006; **7**: 251–260.

CHAPTER 10

Early clinical interventions and outcomes

Louise A. Baur[1,2]

[1] Discipline of Paediatrics & Child Health, University of Sydney, Australia
[2] Weight Management Services, The Children's Hospital at Westmead, Westmead, Australia

Introduction

Childhood obesity is a prevalent health concern in many countries, and thus effective treatment of those affected by obesity is vital. In this chapter, a short overview of the clinical assessment of the obese young child is provided, followed by a review of lifestyle interventions used in treating the obese child in the context of his or her family. Finally, there is a brief consideration of possible child protection issues that may be raised when treating some young children with severe obesity.

Clinical assessment and outcomes

Overweight and particularly obese children present more frequently to primary, secondary and tertiary level clinical services than would be expected from the background prevalence of the condition [1–4]. However, it is rare for obesity to be the main reason for clinical presentation, and, unfortunately, it is also unlikely that the issue will even be raised or addressed by the clinician [1–4] (see Chapter 6). This situation highlights the importance of regular monitoring of height and weight by clinicians and the need for sensitive discussion of concerns about weight issues [5–8].

Clinical assessment

The clinical history should aid in assessing obesity-associated complications and co-morbidities, as well as modifiable lifestyle practices [5–8] (Table 10.1). Physical examination is used to assess obesity-associated co-morbidities and to identify signs of underlying genetic or endocrine disorders. The level of subsequent laboratory investigation, if any, is dependent on the patient's age, severity of obesity, clinical findings and associated familial risk factors. Further discussion of most of these issues is beyond the scope of this review, and readers are referred to national clinical practice guidelines for more information [5–8].

Early Years Nutrition and Healthy Weight, First Edition. Edited by Laura Stewart and Joyce Thompson.
© 2015 John Wiley & Sons, Ltd. Published 2015 by John Wiley & Sons, Ltd.

Table 10.1 Elements of a clinical history in obese children.

General history	Prenatal and birth – history of gestational diabetes and birth weight
	Infant feeding – duration of breastfeeding, timing of introduction of solids
	Current medications – glucocorticoids, some anti-psychotics and anti-epileptics
Weight history	Onset of obesity and duration of parental and child concerns, if any, about the weight
	Previous weight-related interventions
	Previous and current dieting behaviours
Complications history	Psychological – bullying, poor self-esteem, depression
	Sleep – snoring, symptoms suggestive of sleep apnoea
	Exercise tolerance
	Specific symptoms related to gastro-oesophageal reflux, gallstones, orthopaedic complications, enuresis, constipation, benign intracranial hypertension
	Menstrual history (older girls)
Family history	Ethnicity
	Family members with a history of obesity, type 2 diabetes, gestational diabetes, cardiovascular disease, dyslipidaemia, obstructive sleep apnoea, polycystic ovary syndrome, bariatric surgery, eating disorders
Lifestyle history	Diet and eating behaviours – breakfast consumption, snacking, fast-food intake, beverage consumption, family routines around food, binge-eating, sneaking food
	Sedentary behaviour – daily screen time; numbers of TVs, gaming consoles, computers and smart phones in the bedroom and home; pattern of screen time
	Physical activity – play-time, after-school and weekend recreation, sports participation, transport to and from school, family activities
	Sleep – duration and routines

Anthropometry

Body mass index (BMI; weight/height^2) is a clinically useful measure of total body fatness. Height and weight should be measured precisely and accurately, and BMI calculated and then plotted on nationally recommended BMI-for-age charts (see Chapter 3). The specific cut-off points that are used to denote overweight and obesity are somewhat arbitrary and may vary between countries. For example, in the UK, the cut-off points for clinical overweight and obesity are the 91st and 98th percentiles, respectively, compared with the 85th and 95th in the USA, with both using different BMI-for-age charts [5, 7, 8]. Hence, local recommendations should be checked.

Just as in adults, a central fat distribution in children is associated with an increase in cardio-metabolic risk. Waist circumference-for-age charts are available in some countries [9, 10], although no clear-cut points that distinguish between higher and lower risk have been established. A waist circumference to height ratio greater than 0.5 is associated with increased cardio-metabolic risk in school-aged children, is easy to calculate and is not dependent upon access to suitable charts [6, 11, 12]. Importantly, serial measurements of weight, waist and height allow progress to be followed.

Markers of outcome success

When treating a child with obesity, the goals of therapy should be clarified initially with the parents. Markers of a successful outcome of therapy may include improvements in a range of obesity-conducive behaviours, in obesity-associated complications and/or in measures of adiposity, as summarised in Table 10.2. In the still-growing child, a reduction in the rate of weight gain, or weight maintenance, may be the most achievable goal

Table 10.2 Measures of outcome success in childhood obesity.

Improvements in obesity-conducive behaviours	Improvements in obesity-associated complications	Improvements in measures of adiposity
Improvements in: • Eating behaviours, e.g. eating breakfast, drinking water, family meal-times, reduced snacking, regular meals, improved healthy food choices • Physical activity behaviours, e.g. more active transport, regular outdoor play, family recreation time • Sedentary behaviours, e.g. reduced screen time, less passive transport • Sleep duration and patterns • Family functioning and parental oversight of healthy-lifestyle behaviours	• Improved self-esteem and psychosocial functioning • Resolution or appropriate treatment of medical complications, e.g. sleep apnoea, hypertension, insulin resistance, pre-diabetes, dyslipidaemia, fatty liver disease • Increase in level of fitness or aerobic capacity	• Slowing in rate of weight gain • Weight maintenance • Weight loss • Decrease in waist circumference and waist to height ratio

[5–8]. In effect, pre-pubertal children with mild obesity may, over time, be able to 'grow into' an appropriate weight for height. Nevertheless, for moderately to severely obese children, a goal of weight loss will usually be necessary.

Treatment strategies

Overview

Systematic reviews of childhood obesity show that behavioural lifestyle interventions can lead to positive outcomes in weight, BMI and other measures of body fatness [13–15]. This is the case for both the adolescent and pre-adolescent age groups. Improvements in a range of cardio-metabolic risk markers are also seen, although such studies have largely focussed on adolescents rather than on younger children [14]. Further analyses show that the longer the duration of treatment, the greater the observed weight loss [14]. While there is no evidence to support one specific treatment programme over another, meta-analyses show that, in pre-adolescent children, family-targeted behavioural lifestyle interventions can lead to a mean BMI reduction of approximately 1.0kg/m^2 when compared with no treatment/wait list control or usual care [14].

There have been very few treatment trials of overweight or obese children in the first few years of life. In a systematic review of weight management schemes for children aged under 5 years, incorporating papers published up to February 2009, *no studies* aimed at the treatment of overweight or obesity in this age group were identified [16]. A subsequent review of treatment studies of obese children aged 2–7 years that had been published up to August 2011 identified nine randomised controlled trials (RCTs) [15]. Most of these were in primary-school-aged children, rather than in pre-school-aged children, and almost all reported positive weight outcomes. The majority of interventions ($n=7$) targeted parents as the 'exclusive agents of change' and all had at least a moderate intensity (i.e. weekly or more frequent) of face-to-face sessions for part of their programme.

Following this review, the Groningen Expert Center for Kids with Obesity (GECKO) Outpatients Study, conducted in the Netherlands, was published [17]. This RCT involved 75 overweight or obese children aged 3–5 years who were randomised to receive either a 16-week multidisciplinary intervention or usual care. The intervention was reasonably intense, requiring attendance at 25 sessions (dietitian, group physical activity or group behavioural) over the 16-week period. At the end of the 16 weeks, those children in the intervention showed greater decreases in BMI and waist circumference than those in the usual care group. These differences were still evident at 12 months from baseline.

Despite the relative paucity of studies in young children, the key elements of obesity treatment in this age group are well described [5–8, 13, 14]: family engagement, long-term behavioural change, dietary change, increased physical activity, decreased sedentary behaviours, improving sleep pattern and duration, and long-term weight maintenance strategies (see Table 10.3). While many of the studies addressing these

Table 10.3 Key elements of obesity treatment in young children.

Key elements	Possible strategies
Family engagement	Parents as the 'exclusive agents of change'
	Parental role-modelling
	Whole-of-family lifestyle changes
	Focus therapy session on the parents
Long-term behavioural change	Goal setting
	Stimulus control
	Regular monitoring
Dietary change	Regular meals
	Eating together as a family
	Nutrient-rich foods which are lower in energy and glycaemic index
	Increased vegetable and fruit intake
	Healthy snack food options
	Decreased portion sizes
	Water as the main beverage
	Reduction in sugary drink intake
Increased physical activity	Outdoor play
	Incidental activity, e.g. learning to do chores around the home
	Active transport options
	Organised activities for slightly older children
	Improved access to recreation spaces and play equipment
	Involvement in pre-school programmes
Decreased sedentary behaviours	Limit time on the TV, computer, play-station, tablets, smart phones and other small-screens
	<2 years: No screen time
	2–5 years: 1 hour/day
	>5 years: Maximum of 2 hours/day
	Explore alternatives to motorised transport
Improved sleep patterns	Regular bedtime routines, with 'wind-down' time
	Minimise small screen/technology exposure prior to bedtime
	Ensure an early bedtime and adequate sleep duration
Long-term weight maintenance strategies	Family self-management, with therapist support
	Regular monitoring
	Explore phone counselling and internet support options

elements have been undertaken in school-aged children, they are readily applicable, if not more so, to younger children.

Key elements of treatment

Family engagement

There is abundant evidence that family-based interventions can lead to long-term relative weight loss, that is from 2 to 10 years [5–8, 13, 14]. In particular, parental involvement when managing obese pre-adolescent children is vital [5–8, 18, 19]. Most clinical practice guidelines or consensus statements on the management of paediatric obesity highlight the importance of parental and family involvement, although few provide age-specific recommendations [20].

The first study to emphasise the need for a parent-focussed intervention randomised obese children aged 6–11 years and their parents to either parent-only group sessions (highlighting general parenting skills) or child-only group sessions [19, 21]. Both at 1 year and 7 years from baseline, there were significant reductions in overweight in the parent-only group compared with the child-only group. Indeed, at the 7 year follow-up, 60% of the children in the parent-only group versus 31% of those in the child-only group were classified as non-obese [21].

The findings from such studies make developmental sense, as parents/carers should be in charge of the family food and physical activity environments, and should also role model healthy behaviours. The implication for clinical practice is that when treating an obese young child, sessions involving the parent or parents alone, without the young child being present, may be the most effective. Practically, this may mean that the child only attends some sessions and even then is only seen briefly (e.g. for measurement of weight and height) before the parent-focussed part of the therapy occurs.

Behavioural change strategies

Most childhood obesity treatment trials include a behavioural component, often addressing eating, physical activity, sedentary behaviours and, more recently, sleep patterns. Unfortunately, such strategies are often inadequately described [13]. Nevertheless, the use of a greater range of behavioural modification techniques by parents (in the case of younger children) is associated with improved weight outcomes [22]. Some key behavioural change strategies include goal setting, stimulus control and self-monitoring; these were used in most of the studies included in the 2009 Cochrane review of obesity treatment [13].

In goal setting, parents will usually focus upon performance goals (such as changing eating or activity behaviours), although outcome goals (such as specific weight loss) may also be used. An example of a well-specified goal is: *I will not buy any soft drinks or snack foods when I shop each week. To make it easier to do so, I will shop on my own. If the children ask for soft drink, I will offer them water instead, and if they ask for junk food, I will offer fruit or tell them to wait till dinner time.* Considerable time may be needed to help parents set and review behavioural change strategies.

In stimulus control, the parent will modify or restrict environmental influences on eating, physical activity or sleep patterns, in order to facilitate weight control. Examples include removing televisions (TVs) and other screens from bedrooms, using smaller plates and cups at meal times and not storing unhealthy food choices in the house [23].

Self-monitoring, or parental-monitoring in the case of young children, involves the regular recording of a specific behaviour – these records can then be reviewed during clinic visits. Examples may include a daily TV or screen use diary, the daily use of a pedometer to measure aspects of physical activity, a food diary, a sleep pattern diary and weekly weighing. The latter has been shown to aid weight control in treatment-seeking obese adolescents [24] and may be useful when dealing with obese young children and their families.

The variety of communication technologies provides an opportunity to deliver behavioural modification strategies in new ways. For example, short message service (SMS) texts may prompt parental behaviours by acting as a reminder, or parents can send replies to therapist-initiated questions, making simple monitoring easier. Internet monitoring, such as completing sleep or food diaries online, is also possible, as is email communication between parent and therapist. Such strategies are yet to be evaluated for use in families with young obese patients, and hence guidelines are not as yet available.

Dietary change

Dietary change is vital in order to achieve weight control in obese children, although no one dietary prescription appears necessarily superior to another [14, 25]. A 2013 systematic review of dietary and exercise interventions to treat paediatric obesity included several trials in pre-adolescent children, although none in very young children [25]. Most studies used a calorie restriction approach, with varying combinations of macronutrients. Others used the Traffic Light Diet where foods are colour-coded on the basis of nutritional value and energy content to indicate those to be eaten freely (green) or more cautiously (amber, red), or provided general dietary advice. All of the described dietary approaches may lead to sustained weight loss in different settings and age groups [25]. At present, the specific role of dietary macronutrient modification in the management of obese children remains unclear.

In general, dietary interventions should follow national nutrition guidelines and have an emphasis on the following [5–8, 23, 26, 27]:
- regular meals
- eating together as a family, without the TV being on
- choosing nutrient-rich foods which are lower in energy and glycaemic index
- increased vegetable and fruit intake
- healthy snack options
- decreased portion sizes
- drinking water as the main beverage
- a reduction in sugary drink intake
- involvement of the entire family in making sustainable changes to a healthy dietary intake

Increased physical activity

As with dietary modification, changes in child and family physical activity routines will aid weight control and promote health. For example, in obese children aged 8–12 years at baseline, involvement in a 'lifestyle' exercise programme (e.g. walking, cycling, swimming, running, according to preference) is associated with improved weight outcomes at 6 and 17 months when compared with a programme of isocaloric aerobic exercise [28]. A 2006 systematic review showed that in primary-school-aged children and adolescents with obesity, 155–180 minutes/week of supervised moderate-to-high intensity physical activity (with or without a concurrent dietary change) leads to a modest reduction in body fat, although the effects on body weight and abdominal adiposity were inconclusive [29]. The review concluded that there was insufficient evidence to determine the role of isolated or adjunctive weight training.

When working with young children, what strategies can be used to promote increased physical activity [5–8, 13, 23, 25, 27]? In general, these should follow national physical activity guidelines [30, 31] and include the following:
- encouragement of frequent play, particularly outdoor play
- promotion of active transport, for example walking, cycling, using public transport
- promotion of incidental activity, for example helping with household chores
- activities which the child enjoys and which will be sustainable in the long term
- organised exercise or sport programmes have a role particularly in primary-school-aged children – issues of access and sustainability may need to be addressed
- consideration of enrolment in pre-school or in an after-school activity programmes
- involvement of the entire family in making sustainable changes to a healthy level of physical activity

Decreased sedentary behaviours

Several clinical and health promotion guidelines and studies address the issue of targeting sedentary behaviours [5–8, 30–32]. In one of the earliest studies on this issue, 90 obese children aged 8–12 years were assigned to different arms of a behavioural weight control programme: either physical activity or sedentary behaviours were targeted, with two different levels of behavioural change being required [32]. There were similar significant improvements in aerobic fitness, body fat percentage and percentage overweight for all treatment arms at 2 years from baseline, indicating the potential benefit of targeting sedentary behaviours.

In treating obese young children, strategies should follow national sedentary behaviour guidelines [5–8, 26, 30, 31] and should include the following:
- parental supervision and monitoring of children's use of electronic media
- parental role-modelling of healthy behaviours
- remove TVs and other electronic media from bedrooms
- restrict time spent watching TV or using other electronic media (DVDs, computers, other electronic games):
  - Children younger than 2 years: no time with electronic media or small screens
  - Children 2–5 years: limit to 1 hour/day
  - Children 5–12 years: limit to 2 hours/day
- avoid restraining or keeping young children inactive for more than 1 hour at a time, except when sleeping

Improving sleep patterns

There is clear epidemiological evidence that young children who have reduced sleep time are at increased risk of subsequent excess weight gain [33]. This raises the possibility that strategies to improve sleep duration and patterns in obese children may aid weight management, even in the absence of co-morbidities such as obstructive sleep apnoea. However, there are as yet no specific studies addressing this issue. Nor is sleep duration or quality specifically mentioned in current obesity management clinical practice guidelines, apart from the link with obstructive sleep apnoea. Thus, in the absence of specific evidence, clinicians should encourage good age-appropriate sleep hygiene and adhere to national guidelines for sleep duration for children [34, 35].

Plan for long-term weight maintenance

There is still a paucity of clinical trials that report weight management outcomes at 2 or more years from baseline [13, 14]. Nevertheless, in the few that have done so, there are encouraging findings, with many participants maintaining weight reduction outcomes at 2–10 years from baseline without additional intervention [13, 14, 36–38]. It is possible, however, that this may represent a publication bias.

Studies in adults suggest that weight loss maintenance strategies are required for long-term success [6]. A 2007 study addressed this issue in 7–12-year-old obese children [39]. The children underwent an initial 5 month weight management intervention, followed by randomisation to one of three arms: control, 4 months of behavioural skills maintenance or 4 months of social facilitation maintenance treatment. At 2 years from baseline, children in the two maintenance treatment arms had reduced weight regain compared with the control group. Results such as this suggest that a range of strategies needs to be investigated to support longer-term effectiveness of initial weight interventions even in younger children. At present, however, the evidence to guide the nature and type of weight maintenance interventions in this age group is limited. Based on the evidence from adult studies, they are likely to include approaches to support family self-management, continued monitoring by health professionals, and phone counselling and internet support interventions [6].

Challenges in providing clinical services to obese children

One of the difficulties in adapting the existing evidence on obesity treatment to 'real-life' obesity treatment clinics is that such clinics are usually far less well resourced than those in funded clinical trials and may not have a full complement of experienced nursing, allied health or medical staff. In addition, clinic patients may be different from those who participate in clinical trials. For example, they may be more socially disadvantaged, or they or their parents may have a broader range of psychological or medical co-morbidities, thus making engagement in treatment plans more difficult. Table 10.4 outlines some of the potential challenges that may be encountered, and some suggested strategies for tackling them.

Child protection issues and severe obesity

Are there circumstances in which cases of severe obesity in early childhood could give rise to child protection concerns? Paediatric clinicians who treat obese children need to reflect upon this issue, not least because, in many countries, they are required by their state or national laws to report concerns about child protection issues to the relevant child protection authorities. At the same time, it can be difficult to discuss this broad issue in public settings as it is emotive, and there have been dramatic instances of media voyeurism and misreporting [40].

In 1989, two US paediatricians reported 12 cases of severe obesity (ideal body weight for height >150%) in children aged less than 4 years at first presentation, where family psychosocial stress was seen to be critical to the development of obesity [41]. The authors noted several features that were similar to those seen in families where young children had growth failure of psychosocial origin ('failure to thrive'). These included severe family disorganisation, displacement of child care to others, episodic separation of mother and child, maternal depression, ineffective limit-setting, denial of the problem, hostility towards healthcare professionals and inconsistent follow-up with

Table 10.4 Challenges, and possible strategies, in managing childhood obesity in 'real-life' clinical settings.

Challenge and effect	Potential intervention strategy
Clinical service has inadequate staffing to cope with patient load and needs	Review referral criteria Investigate shared care arrangements (e.g. with family doctor, allied health professionals, community nurses) Group programmes Online resources and simple training, to upskill other health professionals
Poverty: Limited access to activities and recreation space Limited access to healthy food choices	Focus on low-cost food options Provision of low-cost physical activity alternatives
Culturally and linguistically diverse patients: Service may not be provided in their first language Cultural practices may not fit with standard advice on diet and activity	Use of interpreters Culturally sensitive weight management advice
Learning disabilities or developmental disorders: Limited ability to benefit from education about diet and activity	Greater family involvement Intensive practical intervention Involvement of specialist support services
Family in crisis (e.g. domestic violence): Child or family is at risk and unable to focus on weight management	Crisis intervention Case management until the situation stabilises Involvement of additional support services such as child protection or social work
Parent has a major psychiatric disorder: Unable to attend treatment or focus on weight management At risk	Involvement of mental health treatment and support services Case management until the situation stabilises
Physical health problems: May not be able to participate in physical activity due to functional limitations	Provide alternative options

medical care. Very severe childhood obesity was conceptualised as being the 'mirror image of failure to thrive', with the authors suggesting that recognisable patterns of family dysfunction were core to the cases they presented. They commented that in these cases of 'severe obesity of psychosocial origin', dietary management alone was 'likely to be useless', primary management needed to be directed towards addressing the psychological issues and social environment, and consideration may need to be given to the removal of the child from the home environment.

It took 20 years before commentaries on this issue began to emerge. In 2009, an Australian group asked whether severe childhood obesity could be considered a form of neglect, and in particular *medical neglect*, that is, where the parent neglects the child's medical needs [42]. Some subsequent reports have stressed that appropriate use of foster care may be required in selected cases [43, 44].

Suggested framework

A UK paper [45] has provided a useful suggested framework for understanding child protection concerns with obese children, highlighting that:

- childhood obesity *alone* is not a child protection issue;
- failure to reduce overweight *alone* is not a child protection issue;

- consistent failure to change lifestyle and engage with outside support indicates neglect, particularly in younger children;
- obesity may be part of wider concerns about neglect or emotional abuse, and
- assessment should include systemic (family and environmental) factors.

Clearly this is a complex and sensitive issue, and clinicians with concerns about individual patients should discuss these with local child protection specialists.

CASE STUDY

CP is a 3-year, 6-month-old boy of Indian ethnic origin who was referred by his family doctor to a multidisciplinary paediatric obesity clinic for management of his obesity. At the time of presentation, his weight was 25.4 kg (99th centile for age; weight-for-age z-score 3.69), height 102.5 cm (84th centile for age; height-for-age z-score 1.01), BMI 24.1 kg/m² (100th centile for age; BMI-for-age z-score 4.43) and waist circumference 66 cm.

His birth weight was 3.93 kg. There were no significant perinatal risk factors and no significant health issues in infancy. He had been breastfed for 18 months. On review of previous growth charts, CP's weight had always been above the 95th centile for age. In terms of social history, CP was the only child of his parents (30-year-old mother, a school teacher; and 37-year-old father, a commercial salesman). He attended day care 3 days/week where he was given lunch. There was a family history, in second-degree relatives, of type 2 diabetes (three grandparents), obesity (maternal grandparents) and hypertension (two grandparents).

Diet history revealed that he was having 600 ml of full cream milk in a bottle, and three to four cups of juice per day. His diet was mainly traditional southern Indian food, with large portions of rice. His parents ate a relatively limited range of foods, with CP's repertoire being even more restricted. He had a low intake of vegetables. CP watched TV up to 6 hours/day, except on days when at day care (2 hours/day).

CP's parents attended a three-session group programme for parents where behavioural lifestyle strategies were introduced. They then had individual appointments with a team of therapists (dietitians, clinical psychologist, nurse, paediatrician, physiotherapist) which were initially offered every 2 weeks, and then became less frequent. In particular, the dietitian encouraged the parents to explore new foods and to be role models for their son. Specific strategies included:

(a) having set meal times and snacks;
(b) ensuring recommended (i.e. smaller) portion sizes so that all meals were lower in carbohydrate;
(c) always offering vegetables as separate dishes;
(d) the parents themselves trying new foods;
(e) the parents being consistent in their approach;
(f) increasing low-fat dairy foods so that calcium intake met recommended intake.

Other strategies that the parents were advised, with support from team members, included:

(a) encouraging parents to spend time playing with CP;
(b) helping parents learn how to play active games with CP, for example squatting games, animal walks, rolling and bouncing a big ball, kicking soccer goals;
(c) offering several activities when CP is 'tired' (i.e. bored);
(d) limiting TV time to an hour per day;
(e) exploring creative play options with the parents.

The parents were also asked to record CP's weight on a weekly basis at home.

The parents were engaged in the treatment programme and attended regularly. They were able to reduce TV time considerably and instituted several of the suggested dietary changes, although CP remained very fussy with his food and there were occasional food battles. At 2 months from initial presentation, CP's weight had decreased to 24.1 kg, with height 103.5 cm, BMI 22.5 kg/m² and waist circumference 64 cm. At 6 months, at the age of 4 years, CP's weight was 23.5 kg (z-score 2.68), height 106.0 cm, BMI 20.9 kg/m² and waist circumference 62.5 cm.

TAKE HOME MESSAGES

- Plot BMI routinely on a BMI-for-age chart.
- Successful outcomes in obese children include improvements in healthy lifestyle behaviours, in obesity-associated complications and/or in measures of body fatness.
- The key elements of obesity management include family engagement, long-term behavioural change, long-term dietary change, increased physical activity, decreased sedentary behaviours, improved sleep patterns and planning for long-term healthy weight maintenance.
- In cases of severe childhood obesity, consider the possibility of child protection concern if there is consistent failure to change lifestyle and engage with outside support.

References

1 Benson L, Baer HJ, Kaelber DC. Trends in the diagnosis of overweight and obesity in children and adolescents: 1999–2007. *Pediatrics* 2009; **123**: 153–158.

2 Cretikos MA, Valenti L, Britt HC, *et al*. General practice management of overweight and obesity in children and adolescents in Australia. *Med Care* 2008; **4**: 1163–1169.

3 Woo JG, Zeller MH, Wilson K, *et al*. Obesity identified by discharge ICD-9 codes underestimates the true prevalence of obesity in hospitalized children. *J Pediatr* 2009; **154**: 327–331.

4 Wake M, Campbell MW, Turner M, *et al*. How training affects paediatricians' management of obesity: Australian national survey linked with prospective practice audit. *Arch Dis Child* 2013; **98**: 3–8.

5 Barlow SE on behalf of the Expert Committee. Expert committee recommendations regarding the prevention, assessment, and treatment of child and adolescent overweight and obesity: summary report. *Pediatrics* 2007; **120** (Suppl 4): 164–192.

6 National Health and Medical Research Council. *Clinical practice guidelines for the management of overweight and obesity in adults, adolescents and children in Australia*. http://www.nhmrc.gov.au/_files_nhmrc/publications/attachments/n57_obesity_guidelines_131204_0.pdf (accessed 1 March 2014).

7 National Institute for Health and Clinical Excellence. *Obesity: guidance on the prevention, identification, assessment and management of overweight and obesity in adults and children. NICE Clinical Guideline 43*. http://guidance.nice.org.uk/CG43/NICEGuidance/pdf/English (accessed 1 March 2014).

8 Scottish Intercollegiate Guidelines Network. *Management of obesity: a national clinical guideline*. http://www.sign.ac.uk/pdf/sign115.pdf/ (accessed 1 March 2014).

9 McCarthy HD, Jarrett KV, Crawley HF. The development of waist circumference percentiles in British children aged 5.0–16.9 y. *Eur J Clin Nutr* 2001; **55**: 902–907.

10 Fernandez JR, Redden DT, Pietrobelli A, *et al*. Waist circumference percentiles in nationally representative samples of African-American, European-American, and Mexican-American children and adolescents. *J Pediatr* 2004; **145**: 439–444.

11 Mokha JS, Srinivasan SR, Dasmahapatra P, *et al*. Utility of waist-to-height ratio in assessing the status of central obesity and related cardiometabolic risk profile among normal weight and overweight/obese children: the Bogalusa Heart Study. *BMC Pediatr* 2010; **10** (73): 1–7.

12 Garnett SP, Baur LA, Cowell CT. Waist to height ratio: a simple option for determining excess central adiposity in young people. *Int J Obes* 2008; **32**: 1028–1030.

13 Oude Luttikhuis H, Baur L, Jansen H, *et al*. Interventions for treating obesity in children. *Cochrane Database Syst Rev* 2009; **1**: CD001872.

14 Ho M, Garnett SP, Baur L, *et al*. Effectiveness of lifestyle interventions in child obesity: systematic review with meta-analysis. *Pediatrics* 2012; **130**: 1647–1671.

15 Knowlden AP, Sharma M. Systematic review of family and home-based interventions targeting paediatric overweight and obesity. *Obes Rev* 2012; **13**: 499–508.

16 Bond M, Wyatt K, Lloyd J, *et al*. Systematic review of the effectiveness of weight management schemes for the under fives. *Obes Rev* 2010; **12**: 242–253.

17 Bocca G, Corpelejin E, Stolk RO, *et al*. Results of a multidisciplinary treatment program in 3-year-old to 5-year-old overweight or obese children: a randomized controlled trial. *Arch Pediatr Adolesc Med* 2012; **166**: 1179–1181.

18 Sung-Chen P, Sung YW, Zhao X, *et al*. Family-based models for childhood-obesity intervention: a systematic review of randomized controlled trials. *Obes Rev* 2013; **14**: 265–278.

19 Golan M, Weizman A, Apter A, *et al.* Parents as the exclusive agents of change in the treatment of childhood obesity. *Am J Clin Nutr* 1998; **67**: 1130–1135.

20 Shrewsbury VA, Steinbeck KS, Torvaldsen S, *et al.* The role of parents in pre-adolescent and adolescent overweight and obesity treatment: a systematic review of clinical recommendations. *Obes Rev* 2011; **12**: 759–769.

21 Golan M, Crow S. Targeting parents exclusively in the treatment of childhood obesity: long-term results. *Obes Res* 2004; **12**: 357–361.

22 McLean N, Griffin S, Toney K, *et al.* Family involvement in weight control, weight maintenance and weight-loss interventions: a systematic review of randomised trials. *Int J Obes* 2003; **27**: 987–1005.

23 Dietz WH, Robinson TN. Clinical practice. Overweight children and adolescents. *N Engl J Med* 2005; **352**: 2100–2109.

24 Saelens BE, McGrath AM. Self-monitoring adherence and adolescent weight control efficacy. *Child Health Care* 2003; **32**: 137–152.

25 Ho M, Garnett SP, Baur LA, *et al.* Impact of dietary and exercise interventions on weight change and metabolic outcomes in obese children and adolescents: a systematic review and meta-analysis of randomised controlled trials. *JAMA Pediatr* 2013; **167**: 759–768.

26 Whitaker RC. Obesity prevention in pediatric primary care: four behaviors to target. *Arch Pediatr Adolesc Med* 2003; **157**: 725–727.

27 Papadaki A, Lindarkis M, Larsen TM, *et al.* The effect of protein and glycemic index on children's body composition: the DiOGenes randomized study. *Pediatrics* 2010; **126**: 1143–1152.

28 Epstein LH, Wing RR, Koeske R, *et al.* A comparison of lifestyle change and programmed exercise on weight and fitness changes in obese children. *Behav Ther* 1982; **13**: 651–665.

29 Atlantis E, Barnes EH, Singh MA. Efficacy of exercise for treating overweight in children and adolescents: a systematic review. *Int J Obes* 2006; **30**: 1027–1040.

30 Australian Government Department of Health. *Australia's physical activity and sedentary behaviour guidelines.* http://www.health.gov.au/internet/main/publishing.nsf/content/health-pubhlth-strateg-phys-act-guidelines (accessed 1 March 2014).

31 United Kingdom Government. *UK physical activity guidelines.* https://www.gov.uk/government/publications/uk-physical-activity-guidelines (accessed 1 March 2014).

32 Epstein LH, Paluch RA, Gordy CC, *et al.* Decreasing sedentary behaviours in treating pediatric obesity. *Arch Pediatr Adolesc Med* 2000; **154**: 220–226.

33 Carter PJ, Taylor BJ, Williams SM, *et al.* Longitudinal analysis of sleep in relation to BMI and body fat in children: the FLAME study. *BMJ* 2011; **342** (2712): 1–7.

34 National Heart, Blood and Lung Institute. *How much sleep is enough?* http://www.nhlbi.nih.gov/health/health-topics/topics/sdd/howmuch.html (accessed 1 March 2014).

35 National Health Service. *How much sleep do kids need?* http://www.nhs.uk/Livewell/Childrenssleep/Pages/howmuchsleep.aspx (accessed 1 March 2014).

36 Epstein LH, Valoski A, Wing RR, *et al.* Ten-year follow-up of behavioral, family-based treatment for obese children. *JAMA* 1990; **264**: 2519–2523.

37 Magarey AM, Perry RA, Baur L, *et al.* A parent-led family-focused treatment program for overweight 5–9 year olds: the PEACH RCT. *Pediatrics* 2011; **127**: 214–222.

38 Collins CE, Okely AD, Morgan PJ, *et al.* Parent-centered diet modification, child-centered activity or both in obese children: an RCT. *Pediatrics* 2011; **127**: 619–627.

39 Wilfley DE, Stein RI, Saelens BE, *et al.* Efficacy of maintenance treatment approaches for childhood overweight: a randomized controlled trial. *JAMA* 2007; **298**: 1661–1673.

40 Australian Broadcasting Corporation (ABC). *Media Watch. Beat up opportunity 'seized'.* http://www.abc.net.au/mediawatch/transcripts/s2499114.htm (accessed 1 March 2014).

41 Christoffel K, Forsyth B. Mirror image of emotional deprivation: severe childhood obesity of psychosocial origin. *Child Abuse Negl* 1989; **13**: 249–256.

42 Alexander SM, Baur LA, Magnusson R, *et al.* When does severe childhood obesity become a child protection issue? *Med J Aust* 2009; **190**: 136–139.

43 Murtagh L, Ludwig DS. State intervention in life-threatening obesity. *JAMA* 2011; **306**: 206–207.

44 Williams GMG, Bredow M, Barton J, *et al.* Can foster care ever be justified for weight management? *Arch Dis Child* 2014; **99**: 297–299.

45 Viner RM, Roche E, Maguire SA, *et al.* When does childhood obesity become a child protection issue? *BMJ* 2010; **341**: 375–377.

Index

Page numbers in *italics* refer to illustrations; those in **bold** refer to tables